THE MODERN ART OF
HIGH INTENSITY TRAINING

THE MODERN ART OF

AURÉLIEN BROUSSAL-DERVAL
STÉPHANE GANNEAU

HIGH INTENSITY TRAINING

HUMAN KINETICS

Library of Congress Cataloging-in-Publication Data

Names: Broussal-Derval, Aurélien, author. | Ganneau, Stephane, author.

Title: The modern art of high intensity training / Aurélien Broussal-Derval, Stephane Ganneau.

Description: Champaign, IL : Human Kinetics, [2017] | Includes bibliographical references.

Identifiers: LCCN 2016050879 (print) | LCCN 2017000410 (ebook) | ISBN 9781492544999 (print) | ISBN 9781492545002 (ebook)

Subjects: LCSH: Exercise. | Exercise--Physiological aspects. | Physical fitness. | Weight training.

Classification: LCC GV481 .B77 2017 (print) | LCC GV481 (ebook) | DDC 613.7/1--dc23

LC record available at https://lccn.loc.gov/2016050879

ISBN: 978-1-4925-4499-9 (print)

This publication is written and published to provide accurate and authoritative information relevant to the subject matter presented. It is published and sold with the understanding that the author and publisher are not engaged in rendering legal, medical, or other professional services by reason of their authorship or publication of this work. If medical or other expert assistance is required, the services of a competent professional person should be sought.

This book is a revised edition of *Méthode Cross Training*, published in 2015 by 4trainer Editions.

The web addresses cited in this text were current as of December, 2016, unless otherwise noted.

Publication/editing: Nadia Belhadj; **Managing Editor:** Nicole Moore; **Copyeditor:** Bob Replinger; **Permissions Manager:** Dalene Reeder; **Graphic Designers:** Nicolas Moreau (www.graphiste-pro.com), Dawn Sills; **Cover Designer:** Nicolas Moreau (www.graphiste-pro.com); **Photographs:** Stéphane Ouzounoff; **Models:** Céline Hardy and Kevin Caesemaeker; **Illustrations:** Stéphane Ganneau; **Printer:** Versa Press

Human Kinetics books are available at special discounts for bulk purchase. Special editions or book excerpts can also be created to specification. For details, contact the Special Sales Manager at Human Kinetics.

Printed in the United States of America   10 9 8 7 6 5 4 3 2 1

The paper in this book is certified under a sustainable forestry program.

Human Kinetics
Website: www.HumanKinetics.com

United States: Human Kinetics
P.O. Box 5076
Champaign, IL 61825-5076
800-747-4457
e-mail: info@hkusa.com

Canada: Human Kinetics
475 Devonshire Road Unit 100
Windsor, ON N8Y 2L5
800-465-7301 (in Canada only)
e-mail: info@hkcanada.com

Europe: Human Kinetics
107 Bradford Road
Stanningley
Leeds LS28 6AT, United Kingdom
+44 (0) 113 255 5665
e-mail: hk@hkeurope.com

Australia: Human Kinetics
57A Price Avenue
Lower Mitcham, South Australia 5062
08 8372 0999
e-mail: info@hkaustralia.com

New Zealand: Human Kinetics
P.O. Box 80
Mitcham Shopping Centre, South Australia 5062
0800 222 062
e-mail: info@hknewzealand.com

E6969

To all the amazing coaches who inspire me each day,
who gave me opportunities and then guided me:
Frankie Lesage, Jane Bridge, Patrick Roux, Ezio Gamba,
and Christian Derval, my father.

ABD.

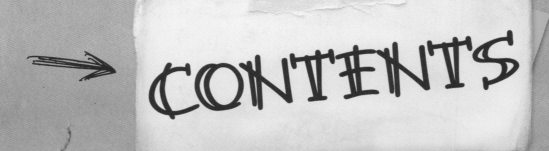

CONTENTS

001   WHY YOU NEED A PROGRAM TO BE SUCCESSFUL

002   TRAINING FUNDAMENTALS AS A STARTING POINT

002   PRINCIPLE 1: PROGRESSION
003   PRINCIPLE 2: CONTINUITY
003   PRINCIPLE 3: VARIETY
003   PRINCIPLE 4: NONLINEARITY
003   PRINCIPLE 5: LOAD AND RECOVERY

004   WHAT YOU SHOULD KNOW ABOUT PHYSIOLOGY

004   THE ENERGY CONTINUUM
004   QUICK, ENERGY!
005   LACTATE IS AT THE HEART OF ENERGY PRODUCTION
006   WHAT ABOUT RECOVERY?
006   ADJUSTING THE INTENSITY
007   USING TIME UNDER TENSION TO ADJUST THE LOAD

008   THINGS THAT INTERFERE WITH TRAINING

008   RULE 1: PRIORITIZE THE WORK
008   RULE 2: WORK OUT IN THE RIGHT ORDER
008   RULE 3: AVOID BAD COMBINATIONS
010   COMBINATIONS THAT WORK

011   HOW TO USE THIS BOOK

012   THE WARM-UP

012   BASIC WARM-UP REMINDERS
014   HOW TO PLAN A WARM-UP
014   Principles to Keep in Mind

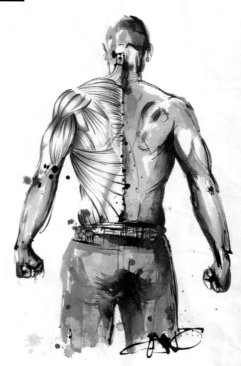

016	**ESSENTIAL PARTS OF THE WARM-UP**
016	(1) General Warm-Up
016	(2) Auxiliary Warm-Up
016	(3) Specific Warm-Up
016	**SPECIFIC HIGH INTENSITY TRAINING ROUTINES**

033   TECHNICAL FOUNDATION

034	**FOUNDATIONAL EXERCISES**
034	**CLEAN AND JERK**
034	**Clean**
046	Workout – Cleans
047	**Jerk**
052	Workout – Jerks
053	Workout – Clean and Jerks
054	**Sandbag Clean**
055	Workout – Sandbags
056	**Tire Clean**
059	Workout – Tire Cleans
060	**Snatch**
075	Workout – Snatches
076	**Kettlebell Variations**
077	Workout – Kettlebell Snatches
082	Workout – Kettlebell Cleans
083	**Bent-Over Row**
088	Workout – Bent-Over Rows

089	**BASIC ATHLETIC EXERCISES**
089	**SQUAT**
089	**Different Types of Squats**
091	**Anatomy Reminders**
092	**How Far Should You Go Down in a Squat?**
093	**Squat Mythology**
093	**Range of Motion and Performance**
095	**Squat Technique**
096	Workout – Squats
097	**Front Squat**
099	Workout – Front Squats

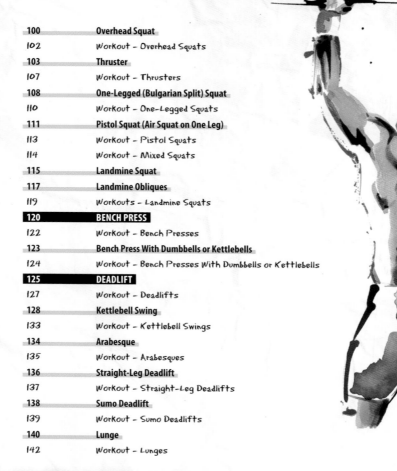

100	**Overhead Squat**
102	*Workout – Overhead Squats*
103	**Thruster**
107	*Workout – Thrusters*
108	**One-Legged (Bulgarian Split) Squat**
110	*Workout – One-Legged Squats*
111	**Pistol Squat (Air Squat on One Leg)**
113	*Workout – Pistol Squats*
114	*Workout – Mixed Squats*
115	**Landmine Squat**
117	**Landmine Obliques**
119	*Workouts – Landmine Squats*
120	**BENCH PRESS**
122	*Workout – Bench Presses*
123	**Bench Press With Dumbbells or Kettlebells**
124	*Workout – Bench Presses With Dumbbells or Kettlebells*
125	**DEADLIFT**
127	*Workout – Deadlifts*
128	**Kettlebell Swing**
133	*Workout – Kettlebell Swings*
134	**Arabesque**
135	*Workout – Arabesques*
136	**Straight-Leg Deadlift**
137	*Workout – Straight-Leg Deadlifts*
138	**Sumo Deadlift**
139	*Workout – Sumo Deadlifts*
140	**Lunge**
142	*Workout – Lunges*
143	**BODYWEIGHT EXERCISES**
143	**FOUNDATION FOR PULL-UPS**
145	*Workout – Pull-Ups*
146	**Archer Pull-Up**
147	*Workout – Archer Pull-Ups*
148	**Open-Hand (Clapping) Pull-Up**
150	*Workout – Clapping Pull-Ups*
153	*Workout – Pull-Ups*
154	**Rope Climbing**
157	*Workout – Ropes*
158	**PUSH-UP**
161	*Workout – Push-Ups*

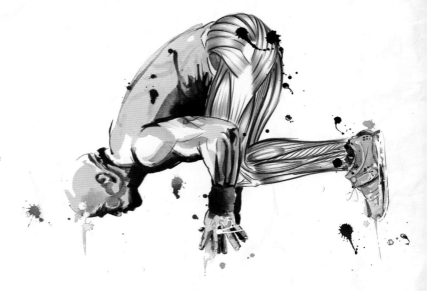

162	**Renegades**
164	*Workout – Renegades*
165	**Burpee**
166	*Workout – Burpees*
167	**Clapping Push-Up**
168	*Workout – Clapping Push-Ups*
169	**EXPLOSIVE PUSH-UP**
169	**Double Knee Tuck Push-Up**
171	**Aztec Push-Up**
172	**Superman Push-Up**
173	*Workout – Explosive Push-Ups*
174	**BATTLE ROPES**
179	*Workout – Battle Ropes*
180	**DIPS**
181	*Workout – Dips*
182	**CORE EXERCISES**
182	**V-Up**
184	*Workout – V-Ups*
185	**Toes to Bar**
186	*Workout – Toes to Bars*
187	**Turkish Get-Up**
189	*Workout – Turkish Get-Ups*
190	**Barbell Ab Rollout**
191	*Workout – Barbell Ab Rollouts*

192   RUNNING

192	**Running Techniques**
193	**A Total-Body Approach to Running Mechanics**
194	**PARAMETERS OF RUNNING**
195	**MECHANICS OF STRIDE ADAPTATION**
198	*Workout – Running*

199   THE 15-WEEK MODERN ART PROGRAM

200	**PHASE 1—FUNDAMENTALS**
202	**PHASE 2—STRUCTURAL DEVELOPMENT**
204	**PHASE 3—INTENSIFY**
206	**PHASE 4—OPTIMIZE**

209   BIBLIOGRAPHY

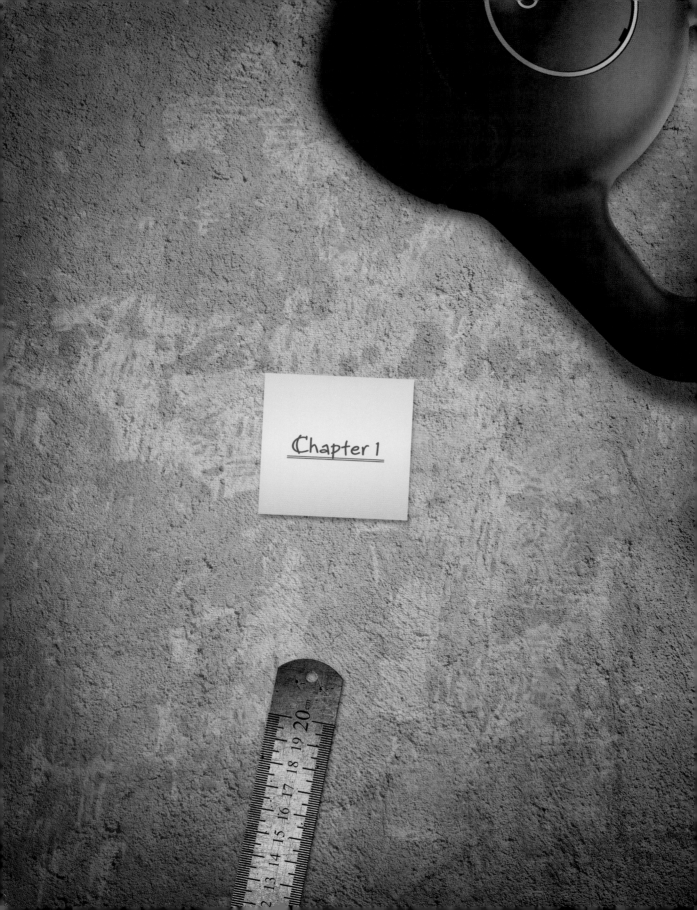

WHY YOU NEED A PROGRAM TO BE SUCCESSFUL

002   Training Fundamentals as a Starting Point

002   Principle 1: Progression
003   Principle 2: Continuity
003   Principle 3: Variety
003   Principle 4: Nonlinearity
003   Principle 5: Load and Recovery

004   What You Should Know About Physiology

004   The Energy Continuum
004   Quick, Energy!
005   Lactate Is at the Heart of Energy Production
006   What About Recovery?
006   Adjusting the Intensity
007   Using Time Under Tension to Adjust the Load

008   Things That Interfere With Training

008   Rule 1: Prioritize the Work
008   Rule 2: Work Out in the Right Order
008   Rule 3: Avoid Bad Combinations
010   Combinations That Work

011   How to Use This Book

012   The Warm-Up
012   Basic Warm-Up Reminders
014   How to Plan a Warm-Up
016   Essential Parts of the Warm-Up
016   Specific High Intensity Training Routines

The greatest asset of high intensity training is also its biggest weakness. The variety inherent in many programs is what attracts most people and holds their interest. But starting a new program that is different and innovative in many ways, using different weights, and doing a new workout daily can lead to counterproductive methods of improvisation. Changing things up, solely for the sake of change, could result in unintended consequences. Obviously, you can vary your training, but there is an art to doing so. What follows within is *The Modern Art of High Intensity Training*.

TRAINING FUNDAMENTALS AS A STARTING POINT

As in any discipline, training is based on fundamental precepts that should never be compromised for any reason, even to keep things new. The training principles follow.

✖ PRINCIPLE 1: PROGRESSION

This principle is based not only on physiology and pedagogy but also on common sense. Some gyms and fitness clubs try to increase membership by promoting challenging but complex routines. These routines highlight a number of tools but ignore the basic concept of progression. This philosophy comes from the idea that participants are coming to the club to feel good and have fun, so the club should give them their money's worth as quickly as possible. First, this view is contrary to the progression required in high intensity training. It separates a person's technical development from his or her physical progress.

The fundamental techniques of common high intensity training exercises are too complex to assume that anyone can master them in an instant. Instead, participants must work for several months to be able to perform exercises efficiently and without risk of injury; success can be achieved only through serious work on the basics.

Specific instruction, especially for the snatch and clean and jerk exercises, is important from the start.

The complexity of high intensity training is not only technical but also physiological. Workouts often require several physical attributes (sometimes these attributes are antagonistic; see the section later in the book devoted to interference in training). The most intense attributes rely on the methodical and gradual development of metabolic endurance, involving basic adaptations without which the effectiveness of future training could be compromised. Of course, you can train every part of your body, but that does not mean you should do it in a random order.

Metabolic endurance, characterized by varying levels of intensity and sustained effort, involves primary physiological adaptations that cannot be developed in other ways (or can only be developed to a lesser degree). Relevant terms here include plasma volume, stroke volume, and the force of left ventricle contraction. If these aspects are not rigorously developed using a suitable program at the beginning, they may limit future progress.

Progression should be evident in any program even though people are often tempted to skip the warm-up. In most clubs, instructors are taught the importance and principles of warming up. But when you add the time required for a gradual, thorough warm-up to the time needed for a complete workout, the standard 60-minute time frame is sometimes not enough. So in practice, the warm-up is often cut short.

Reactivating motor patterns gradually (indeed, training them), becoming psychologically awake, and optimizing physiological parameters will all guarantee a successful workout (see The Warm-Up section starting on page 12 for more information). A warm-up with a gradual increase in weight and exercise complexity creates optimal conditions for the main workout.

✖ PRINCIPLE 2: CONTINUITY

Keep in mind that short-term progress is unstable. To make such progress permanent, you need to continue using consistent loads in a similar pattern over several workouts. In fact, randomly changing programs from one workout to the next means that you will never create lasting adaptations, greatly limiting your potential.

Some exercise classes or training programs rely on the "instant results" fitness approach. But the risk of doing a little of everything is ultimately doing a lot of nothing. This book will show you how to create a functional training program that will deliver real and lasting results.

✖ PRINCIPLE 3: VARIETY

Workout variety increases motivation by continually surprising an athlete and avoiding a boring workout routine. This principle does not necessarily have to conflict with the other principles. It can provide a perfect balance of rigor and variety.

✖ PRINCIPLE 4: NONLINEARITY

Nonlinearity is another basic principle widely associated with high intensity training, especially in the choice of exercises. A purposeful mixture of different types of exercises is arranged in a variety of sequences and has the goal of creating a novel or unusual training stress. Nonlinearity can also be applied to load and volume (sets, times, reps). Instead of the traditional use of gradually progressive blocks of training, nonlinear load and volume changes occur more often (even weekly or daily) within shorter training phases to provide more variation in the training stimulus.

✖ PRINCIPLE 5: LOAD AND RECOVERY

A good reason to take back control of your workout program is to create an optimal balance between load and recovery. Whether you are in the middle of a workout or between two workouts, you should never plan your workload without considering the recovery required.

First, recovery guarantees a return to a fresh state so that the body is again able to perform intense training. Second, most of the progress that results from a workout actually occurs during recovery.

You'll find that our approach is rigorous when it comes to scheduling and managing recovery.

WHAT YOU SHOULD KNOW ABOUT PHYSIOLOGY

You probably already know that muscle is made up of different types of fibers. As a reminder, muscles include slow-twitch and fast-twitch fibers. Slow-twitch fibers are especially vascular and rich in mitochondria. Their maximum performance occurs during repetitive or prolonged contractions at below maximum intensity. In contrast, fast-twitch fibers are the most effective during intense contractions and during short bursts of maximum effort. Fast-twitch fibers can be further divided into two subcategories: fibers that can be easily fatigued and fibers that are somewhat harder to fatigue. The physiology of any effort is subject to these mechanisms of contraction. Physical performance, from a motor standpoint, depends on combining these contractions together. To do this, you need a system to convert fuel into energy.

✱ THE ENERGY CONTINUUM

Depending on the intensity and duration of a workout, the production of energy is accomplished with or without the availability of oxygen. The breakdown of glucose (which is the primary fuel) during exercise continues as the effort is prolonged (and so long as the intensity is kept low enough) by using more and more oxygen. People talk about anaerobic (without oxygen) or aerobic (with oxygen) pathways, but the mechanism is really a continuum in which the dominant pathway depends on the type of physical effort.

The human body is a hybrid motor propelled by several energy-producing systems that take control depending on the situation.

High intensity training is interesting in this context because it oscillates between the aerobic and anaerobic systems through varying levels of intensity throughout the workout. You often hear people discuss lactate in this situation.

✱ QUICK, ENERGY!

When exercise intensity increases and muscle contractions are repetitive and intense, the fast-twitch fibers produce a lot of lactate.

The stored form of glucose, called glycogen, is broken down into pyruvate (which then helps the body produce energy). Pyruvate enters the mitochondria, where, when combined with oxygen, it is transformed into energy (the aerobic pathway). But as intensity increases, the fast-twitch fibers are recruited and the production of pyruvate becomes too much for the mitochondria to handle. Pyruvate builds up at the entrance to the mitochondria and is converted into lactate. This is the anaerobic pathway.

This is what happens in high intensity training circuits. The intensity is high enough that the two systems function together; the accelerated breakdown of glucose required to produce energy for intense muscle contractions results in the production of a large amount of pyruvate. The mitochondria cannot handle too much pyruvate, leading to the production of lactate.

Why lactate is so important

The efficiency with which the body transforms glucose into energy comes, in part, from the ability of the body to liberate glucose by transporting H+ protons. The production of lactate allows the proton transporters to release their cargo and pick up more quickly. So the creation of lactate helps maintain a rapid glucose breakdown flow.

This mechanism helps explain why the more lactate you produce, the more capable you are of an intense effort.

✖ LACTATE IS AT THE HEART OF ENERGY PRODUCTION

As we have already explained, lactate is mostly produced by fast-twitch fibers whose mitochondrial saturation accelerates the production of pyruvate during intense exercise. This process is exactly what happens during high intensity training, which generates a lot of lactate.

Lactate is then captured by the neighboring slow-twitch fibers to be used for energy by the aerobic pathway. Any remaining lactate enters the bloodstream and is used as energy by the heart or by other slow-twitch fibers that become available during active recovery.

For that reason, we use mostly active recovery periods during the workouts.

Extensive capacity and repetitive capacity

In 2007 Aubert and Chauffin identified an **important concept** called repetitive capacity. Before then, energy pathways were understood to be like machines, with both power (maximum intensity produced during effort in a given pathway) and capacity (delay in the time to fatigue of the system in use, which is gradually abandoned in favor of the power of the next system).

It is this second part that the authors called **extensive capacity**. They compare it to repetitive capacity, which is the potential for repetitive, high intensity effort within the same system.

Here we are talking about enduring power, a specific requirement for high intensity training.

Single sets

Since about 2010, a stirring debate has been ongoing about single sets versus multiple sets. Some researchers and coaches promoted the seductive idea that a single set, pushed to failure (the moment when you cannot do another repetition) would be only slightly less effective than multiple sets and that the difference was not great enough to justify doing multiple sets (generally, the single-set myth states that the gain from doing multiple sets is only 3 percent greater).

These theories echoed throughout the high intensity training community, where long, burning sets and short workouts are especially popular.

Even though the majority of studies have since disproved this theory, here are a few final arguments to convince you that four is better than one.

- Who would turn down a 3 percent increase in performance?

- Muscle growth occurs in fatigued muscle fibers following maximum muscle tension. The causes for muscle saturation vary, and a single set can be stopped for other reasons than complete local muscular saturation (e.g., central nervous system fatigue, psychological fatigue, blood acidity, a decrease in energy reserves, and, especially, a lack of technical expertise).

In other words, a set pushed to failure is effective, but these sets should not be used exclusively. Single sets should be combined with other methods for the best results.

As much as possible, maximum effort should be duplicated from one set to the next, illustrating this book's concept of multiple single sets or of a repeated single set.

✱ WHAT ABOUT RECOVERY?

The peak of lactatemia following an intense set comes about 7 minutes after the set ends. The level returns to normal 60 minutes later (not 24 to 48 hours later as is sometimes said). This means that people can do two intense high intensity workouts on the same day or on consecutive days. What is more likely to cause a problem is the accumulation of nervous system and metabolic loads day after day. For that reason, we plan 1 day of rest every 3 days. Furthermore, active recovery at 40 to 50 percent of $\dot{V}O_2$ max (maximum quantity of oxygen that can be used during the exercise) significantly accelerates the removal of lactate from the blood.

We always provide an active recovery sequence of a specified intensity after every prolonged intense exercise.

In 2006, however, Spencer and colleagues taught us that after very intense or even maximum effort over a brief period, passive recovery is better for resynthesizing phosphocreatine. For strength-based workouts and high intensity sprints, our method favors this type of recovery. Note that repeating your maximum effort after a rest period of less than 10 seconds by depleting muscle energy stores (phosphocreatine) may compromise the rest of the workout (decreased intensity, poor technique, or the length of the workout). For that reason, we include these kinds of workouts in our method.

✱ ADJUSTING THE INTENSITY

When working with large groups, a common approach is to recommend a standard weight for the whole group.

In these cases, the workout provides an identical number of repetitions and a defined bar weight for everyone (perhaps adjusted for men, women, and competitive athletes). In a group setting, however, body type varies significantly from one person to the next, even among the same gender and among similar fitness levels. Some athletes may be comfortable at 70 percent of their maximum weight, easily handling a dozen repetitions, whereas a partner, who may have a higher maximum weight, fails after only 10 repetitions.

Another argument focuses on technique. Some people with better technique can economize their movement, so they will need to adjust their weight to make as much progress as beginners make.

A final argument concerns body weight, which can create significant differences in maximum strength but also increases the amount of weight that can be used in certain exercises. For example, the intensity of a squat with 220 pounds (100 kg) depends on both the weight on the bar and the person's body weight. Obviously, the same weight cannot be assigned to a person who weighs 132 pounds (60 kg) and one who weighs 265 pounds (120 kg). This consideration is especially important in pull-ups. Take as an example a beginner who weighs 198 pounds (90 kg); he or she will start training with a supramaximal load for that exercise! The person will need a way to lighten the load. Therefore, the simple instruction "Everyone should do 10 pull-ups" is clearly not enough.

In practice, this means that if a group workout suggests 10 squats with 220 pounds (100 kg) followed by 20 pull-ups done as many times as possible in 5 minutes, each member of that group will experience a very different workout, too different in fact.

Therefore, we suggest more adaptable alternatives:

Sometimes people say that lactic acid limits performance. Now you understand that lactate is, in reality, a precious source of energy.

The factor that is truly responsible for muscle acidosis is the proton produced when glucose is broken down for energy, which leaves the cell at the same time as lactate.

So lactate struggles with intracellular acidosis at the same time it is providing energy!

● We often talk about X-rep max. This term describes the maximum weight that you can lift X times. For example, a five-rep max is the amount of weight you can lift five times before you fail on the sixth rep.

● We will not always specify a weight so that you can choose the best weight for your workout. You should adjust the weight during the workout if you find that it is too heavy or too light.

● Of course, technical adjustments and variations that make the exercise easier are still a powerful tool that people use to customize the weight. This approach will surely continue to be used.

Developing your buffering capacity

The bad reputation of lactate lingers. You still hear too much talk about lactic acid, even though such acid levels do not exist in the human body (lactic acid has a pH of 3.5, but the human body has a pH of about 6.5). The confusion comes in part from acidosis, which regulates adaptations to intense exercise.

On the one hand, lactate promotes adaptation, especially protein synthesis, and on the other hand, protons promote acidity in the environment and protein breakdown.

The key to regulating this antagonistic effect is to develop the body's buffering capacity, which helps neutralize the protons.

Many research studies have tried to determine the most effective way to do this: The buffering capacity of a muscle is dramatically changed after a workout using 2-minute sets at 80 to 90 percent of $\dot{V}O_2$ max intensity with 1-minute rest breaks between sets.

For that reason, during cycles devoted to improving this potential, our method suggests these types of workouts.

✖ USING TIME UNDER TENSION TO ADJUST THE LOAD

Working hard in training does not necessarily mean using heavy weights. Focusing on performing an exercise precisely will instantly make it more challenging. After an athlete progresses, she or he can think of time under tension, measured by the time required for the movement. The act of measuring the time devoted to each phase of a squat is an effective way to increase the effect of a set without increasing the weight or doing a huge number of sets.

As an example, think of the four parts of a squat, all measured in seconds. The first part is standing with straight legs, the next part is the downward movement, the third part is the bottom position (at a variable height depending on the squat), and the last part is the upward movement. Depending on how many seconds you spend in each of these parts of the exercise, you can completely change the workload even when using the same amount of weight. To convince yourself of this, first do a parallel squat at regular speed. Now repeat the exercise without changing the amount of weight but this time take 3 seconds to go down and spend 1 second in the parallel position. You might want to rethink the number of reps you'll do as you are going down!

THINGS THAT INTERFERE WITH TRAINING

The popularity of high intensity training has gone hand in hand with scientists' growing interest in combined workouts. At the beginning of the 2000s, many studies were done on combining different types of training during the same workout or in the same set. Although results vary depending on the fitness level of the athletes and the weight used in the workout, studies agree on a certain number of rules that we will try to apply to our approach.

✱ RULE 1: PRIORITIZE THE WORK

Most studies agree that training programs dedicated to strength will have a greater effect on strength and programs dedicated to cardiovascular endurance will have a greater effect on cardiovascular endurance. We are talking about the limits of the all-in-one approach taken in traditional high intensity training. To achieve real progress, you must keep in mind one of the principles of training: Working out means making choices. Recent studies such as those conducted by Jones and colleagues also remind us that the frequency of cardiovascular endurance training should be low if the primary objective during a given cycle is to develop strength. Without compromising the richness of high intensity training, our approach establishes clear priorities for each cycle and each workout. Therefore, every workout will have a single theme.

✱ RULE 2: WORK OUT IN THE RIGHT ORDER

One idea that comes out of numerous studies, which you can easily find in the bibliography, is the priority of neuromuscular parameters on cardiovascular endurance. In fact, starting a workout with aerobic endurance training always seems to produce less satisfactory results on improving strength than starting with strength training. The stress on the nervous system during the initial aerobic endurance training undoubtedly affects the athlete's ability to generate strength during the subsequent resistance training workout. For those just starting to train, however, Davitt and his team showed that the order of resistance training and aerobic endurance training is irrelevant. After eight weeks of training, significant improvement occurred in muscular strength and cardiovascular endurance, regardless of the order of training.

Whether during the workout or during the day, our approach gives you a plan that emphasizes strength-oriented training sequences. In that case, to optimize potential progress, we recommend that you plan as much recovery time as possible between workouts.

✱ RULE 3: AVOID BAD COMBINATIONS

An important notion brought to light in modern training is interference between incompatible training modes. In high intensity training, in which combined workouts make up the activity, the trick is to limit interference as much as possible by avoiding certain training sequences, not only within the same workout but also within the same cycle. The most representative model is undoubtedly the one proposed by Docherty and Sporer. → *See the diagram on the next page.*

The most antagonistic training sequences are those that combine resistance training (using sets of 8 to 12 RMs) and intermittent aerobic training at high intensity (an intensity close to maximal aerobic power or $\dot{V}O_2$ max). The combination of these two types of sequences, both producing incompatible peripheral effects, should be avoided.

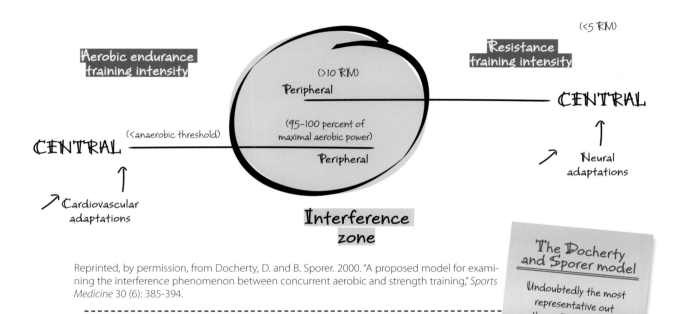

Aerobic endurance training intensity

Resistance training intensity

(<5 RM)

(>10 RM)
Peripheral

CENTRAL

(95-100 percent of maximal aerobic power)

Peripheral

CENTRAL (<anaerobic threshold)

↗ Neural adaptations

↗ Cardiovascular adaptations

Interference zone

Reprinted, by permission, from Docherty, D. and B. Sporer. 2000. "A proposed model for examining the interference phenomenon between concurrent aerobic and strength training," *Sports Medicine* 30 (6): 385-394.

The Docherty and Sporer model

Undoubtedly the most representative out there. Objective: to avoid bad combinations and interference

Why do some high intensity training circuits not work?

The Docherty and Sporer model clearly explains the maximum interference zone that you should absolutely avoid. But some workouts run into problems in precisely this zone. Remember that just because a workout is hard does not mean it is effective!

So working on aerobic endurance through interval training at an intensity close to maximum aerobic power with the goal of increasing the oxidative capacity of the muscles should never be combined with resistance training using sets of 8 to 12 RM loads per exercise. These kinds of sets are used to increase protein synthesis and to generate stress in the anaerobic energy system, which is accompanied by an increase in lactate concentration within the muscle.

The body would have to adjust to two different physiological constraints at the same time, which reduces any potential adaptations in one system or maybe even both.

✖ COMBINATIONS THAT WORK

Appropriate combinations of training sequences cannot be chosen at random! Some combinations work better than others. The best combinations minimize interference within a workout and as much as possible within the entire training program. Here are two examples for guidance that will help you understand how our workouts are organized.

Things to remember about rules for combinations

- Avoid combining exercises using 8 to 12 RM loads with intense cardio sets.
- Do not use a load lighter than an 8 RM for an exercise when the workout combines strength and aerobic power training.
- A good combination is aerobic interval training and maximum strength or power training.
- Low intensity continuous aerobic training can be combined with strength training.

Strength or power training

Very high intensity sets

Strength: 2 to 5 RMs, complete recovery (3 to 5 minutes)

Power: 4 to 6 reps at maximum speed, near-complete recovery (2 to 3 minutes).

Physiological objective: Improve nervous system control

+

High intensity interval training

Sets that are close to maximal aerobic power

Examples:

15 reps x 30 seconds of effort at 105 percent of VO_2 max; then 30 seconds of recovery

10 x 45 seconds of effort at 95 percent of VO_2 max; then 15 seconds of recovery

Physiological objective: Increase the oxidative capacity of the muscles

In this example, by combining strength or power training with high intensity interval training, we are targeting both neural adaptations and oxidative capacity adaptations, which do not interfere with each other much.

Low intensity aerobic endurance training

Continuous exercise at moderate intensity

The work can be done in a circuit but with minimal rest breaks. Sets should be combined with as little rest as possible between sets so that the muscles are worked as continuously as possible. Finally, the workout should be long enough that high intensity intervals are not possible and the aerobic oxidative processes are activated. Workouts should be 12 to 20 minutes long.

Physiological objective: Optimize cardiopulmonary mechanisms

+

Muscle mass and volume training

Sets in which you push close to failure, using maximum weight in longer sets of 8 to 12 RMs

Physiological objective: Muscle hypertrophy

In this example, by combining muscle hypertrophy training with basic aerobic endurance work, we are focusing on both hypertrophy adaptation and cardiopulmonary adaptation, which interfere little with each other.

HOW TO USE THIS BOOK

Please remember that this book cannot be a substitute for a good professional strength coach or personal trainer. It will help reinforce your knowledge, but it is not intended to teach you basic techniques. We assume that readers of this book are seasoned athletes, although a beginner could, in theory, perform these exercises by just reading them. This book may also take you off the beaten path, because it does not always follow conventional training guidelines. We sometimes do things differently to respond better to physiological needs or encourage more progress. Don't be surprised!

If you would like to follow a complete 15-week program, then the section at the end of the book dedicated to that program is made for you. This section provides a clear explanation of workouts that will allow you to make definitive progress, whatever your current level. Of course, you can expand on this plan to suit your needs by following the advice in this book.

If you are an advanced athlete capable of designing your own program, various workouts organized according to theme are offered throughout this book. Note that this approach is not intended to compete with franchises or organized groups. It can complement and enrich them, but you should not abandon quality content available in instructor-led training.

THE WARM-UP

✱ BASIC WARM-UP REMINDERS

A warm-up is a preparatory and preventive activity for the body that happens before effective exercise begins. The warm-up for some programs, however, is often summary, routine, and nonspecific. We need to point out three negative things regarding modern, but basic, warm-up techniques.

Too often, a few minutes of rowing or jumping rope followed by lifting an empty bar serve as the warm-up before the workout. Athletes who are already focused on their workouts often decide to get the warm-up out of the way as quickly as possible so that they can get to work.

Warm-ups may be incomplete (missing a type of work or skipping a part of the body), done out of habit (always doing the same warm-up), or even inappropriate (for the circumstances, for the athlete, or for the content of the workout).

Although warm-up methods are numerous and sometimes similar in conception, even while being total opposites, one concept is always important: elevating the internal temperature of the muscle. In 1979, Bergh and Ekblom noted that maximal strength and power increase as muscle temperature increases.

The increase in strength is about 2 percent per 1.8 °F (1 °C), which, among competitive athletes, could be a determining factor (especially in power lifting and weightlifting, in which 2 percent could translate into a lot more weight!). Because the temperature of the muscles and tendons at rest is about 98.6 °F (37 °C), the goal is to drive that temperature up by doing a warm-up.

At these temperatures, physiological reactions function optimally and the speed of biochemical reactions is at its highest (Schmidt and Thews 2013). If the muscles and tendons are most productive at a temperature of 102.2 °F (39 °C), the same holds true for the nervous system and the joints.

We will now cover the five main effects of a successful warm-up:

→ See the table on the next page.

Things to avoid!

Holding static poses after a general warm-up, which makes you lose all the good effects (for example, running followed by a long series of floor stretches)

- Training circuits done as a warm-up involving a drastic increase in heart rate but no significant change in cardiac output

- Warm-ups that are too long or too short

- Passive stretching used as a warm-up

- Warming up with an ointment, which has only a peripheral effect

- Warming up with sudden, complex motor exercises (weightlifting exercises, kettlebell, and so on)

Elevated internal muscle temperature	Greater cardiac output	Higher respiratory minute volume	Improvement in motor efficiency	Psychological effects
➋ Faster metabolic reactions ➋ Decrease in viscoelastic behavior ➋ Increase in muscle extensibility and decrease in internal tension ➋ Increase in the speed with which the muscle shortens and thus the contraction time ➋ Better muscle excitability ➋ Superior nerve conduction speed ➋ Increase in strength production	➋ Increase in heart rate ➋ Increase in systolic ejection fraction ➋ Better muscle perfusion (to a certain extent) ➋ Decrease in total peripheral resistance (better blood circulation) ➋ Vasodilation of active muscle areas, vasoconstriction of inactive muscle areas (optimization of blood supply as a function of need)	➋ Increase in respiration ➋ Increase in tidal volume ➋ Increase and optimization of pulmonary gas exchange to cause better uptake of O_2 (and energy production) and better removal of CO_2	➋ Improved proprioception (better reaction of the neuromuscular pathways above 100.4 °F [38 °C]) ➋ Protection for joints by thickening of the cartilage (10 percent) ➋ Better joint mobility (increase in intra-articular fluid) ➋ Improvement of muscle synergy ➋ Reactivation of motor patterns by refreshing motor memory (to recover automated movements)	➋ Increased confidence ➋ Increased motivation and preparedness for the harder exercises that make up the workout ➋ Optimized attention and focus

In the intermediate phase between resting and the beginning of intense exercise, a warm-up should

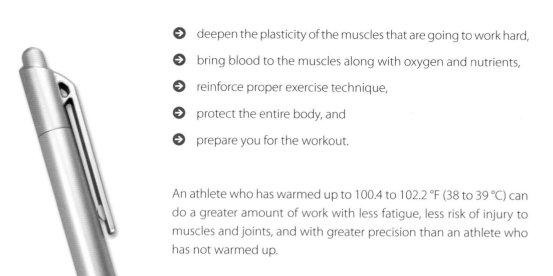

➋ deepen the plasticity of the muscles that are going to work hard,

➋ bring blood to the muscles along with oxygen and nutrients,

➋ reinforce proper exercise technique,

➋ protect the entire body, and

➋ prepare you for the workout.

An athlete who has warmed up to 100.4 to 102.2 °F (38 to 39 °C) can do a greater amount of work with less fatigue, less risk of injury to muscles and joints, and with greater precision than an athlete who has not warmed up.

✖ HOW TO PLAN A WARM-UP

Unfortunately, no single customized warm-up is both perfectly designed around the scientific principles of sport and appropriate for every type of workout.

Forget the dream of an ultimate warm-up routine. The most important aspect is that the warm-up should be adapted to an individual and to the planned workout. Because our workouts can be done any time of the year, anywhere in the world, indoors or outdoors, and because you can work out almost every day, here are the various elements that you should keep in mind to customize your warm-up for any situation:

In the cold (below 57 °F [14 °C])	In the heat (above 68 °F [20 °C])	Time of day	Type of workout planned
➍ Wear appropriate clothing to conserve the heat you generate; otherwise, the warm-up is pointless. Be sure to cover the muscles you are going to work. ➍ Warm up for a little longer to ensure you generate enough heat to raise the internal temperature of your large muscle groups.	➍ Hydrate regularly (before you feel thirsty). ➍ Find a temperate, open-air location for your warm-up (in the shade). ➍ Promote the circulation of fresh air (windows open and using a fan). ➍ Most important, avoid becoming overheated and suffering heatstroke.	➍ Warm-ups done early in the morning or in the evening should be longer and more conscientious than warm-ups done during the day. ➍ Take the athlete's psychological situation into account (for example, personal problems).	➍ For short, maximum intensity workouts, use an in-depth warm-up that does not tire out the body. ➍ In 1972 Stoboy suggested a 15- to 30- minute warm-up (perhaps longer if the type of workout requires it). ➍ For a shorter, high intensity workout, the warm-up should be focused and last for a minimum of 20 minutes. ➍ Finally, for long, low intensity workouts, a brief warm-up (less than 10 minutes) should suffice (Radlinger 1998).

PRINCIPLES TO KEEP IN MIND

A warm-up can be effective and beneficial if you follow these four rules:

➍ **Generate some real heat**: The temperature of the body increases only if the power provided by the muscles is greater than 50 watts, so the intensity has to be high enough. Be careful: The amount that a person sweats varies greatly from one person to another, so perspiration is not a good way to judge a warm-up. Heart rate is a much better indicator: either between 140 and 160 beats per minute or between 60 and 80 percent of functional capacity.

➍ **Conserve the heat**: The body cools down through radiation (the body radiates infrared heat and cools itself) and evaporation (sweating). The cooler the temperature is, the more important it is to wear sufficient clothing.

➍ **Warm up gradually**: Don't exhaust yourself (maintain your energy). The combination of exercises you use should allow you to increase the intensity gradually right up until the beginning of the workout.

➍ **Alternate the work**: It is imperative, both physically and psychologically, to alternate exercises and add variety to your warm-up. You should perform exercises that recruit your cardiorespiratory system as well as exercises that activate different muscle groups and joints. In this way, whole-body and muscle-specific exercises are combined in the warm-up in a varied fashion.

Hamstrings

The function and particular anatomical and physiological structure of the hamstrings warrant a special approach.

The hamstrings are V-shaped, pennate muscles made up of numerous short fibers with a great deal of connective tissue, so they have a strong tendency to be stiff.

From now on, you must be proactive about your hamstrings:

- Warm up first using leg curl variations (opening and closing the feet with pointed or flexed feet) while inclining the torso at various angles and moving the pelvis from a tilted-forward to a tilted-backward position (see photo). →

- After a workout, stretch thoroughly (to restore their original length and maintain the initial eccentric function).

- When using a leg curl machine, remember to alternate the legs so that both sides do equal work.

- Eccentric training, which is more demanding, should be preceded by concentric training (or even isometric training).

- Finish with dynamic leg curls to get the muscles back into their regular movement pattern (and some possible isometric training such as straight-leg running).

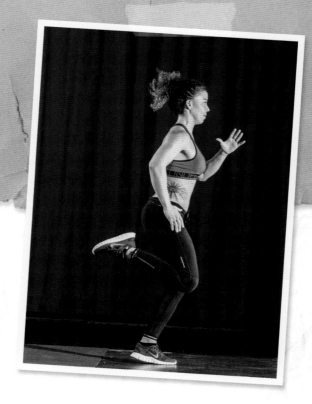

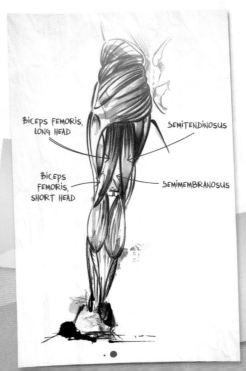

BICEPS FEMORIS, LONG HEAD

SEMITENDINOSUS

BICEPS FEMORIS, SHORT HEAD

SEMIMEMBRANOSUS

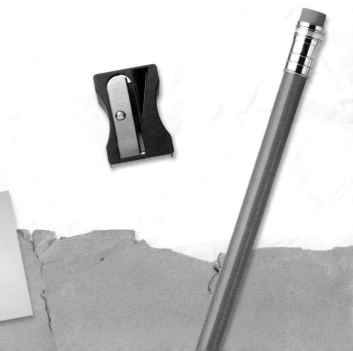

✖ ESSENTIAL PARTS OF THE WARM-UP

A modern warm-up includes three parts that should always be included. The choice of content and length that we provide here are only examples; they are not the ultimate combination! You should select your exercises systematically depending on the context and while following the principles we have already given you.

Be careful! Just 10 to 15 minutes is enough time for your core and your head to reach 102.2 °F (39 °C). Do not trust in that alone, because it will take 10 minutes more for your limbs (and those muscles) to reach 100.4 °F (38 °C) (especially because of greater loss of heat and the difference in blood volume between these areas).

1. GENERAL WARM-UP

Length: 5 minutes

The goal of this part of the warm-up is to activate the cardiopulmonary system by gradually waking up the cardiac and respiratory systems. To do this, the focus should be on low-intensity total-body exercise. Running is perfect for this, provided you remember to include variations (crossing, high knees, and so on).

2. AUXILIARY WARM-UP

Length: 5 to 10 minutes

This part of the warm-up builds on the previous step and consists of alternating exercises while maintaining cardiopulmonary activity:

- Waking up the various joints and exposing them to some tension (especially the neck and the extremities)
- Running again with moderate intensity
- Active dynamic stretches consisting of stretching for about 8 seconds, contracting for about 8 seconds, and then dynamically stretching for about 8 seconds
- Running again with variations for intensity (short sprints)

3. SPECIFIC WARM-UP

Length: 10 minutes (can be combined with the technical content of the actual workout)

Envision your warm-up with the workout in mind. A complete warm-up should include specific components for

- the particular needs of the athlete (a noted weakness or a distinctive need of the athlete's body) and
- the specific requirements of the exercises that will be performed in the workout.

The technical areas are of primary concern: footwork or strides, squats with varying levels of strength, or semitechnical weightlifting exercises.

The last part of the warm-up is the essential transition that leads from a total-body warm-up to the heart of the workout by specifically reactivating the motor patterns and muscle memory.

Here are a few suggestions for specific routines for various kinds of workouts.

✖ SPECIFIC HIGH INTENSITY TRAINING ROUTINES

After you understand the basic principles for the warm-up, and, most important, apply them, you need to master specific movements for the sport to reactivate specific motor patterns and prepare yourself both physically and mentally for the exercises in the workout.

Note that these exercises are suggestions for combinations and could (should!) be enriched, mixed up, and adapted. Finally, we want to clarify that these exercises are as much conditioning and preventive routines as they are educational routines adapted for high intensity training.

Barbell Routine

Exercise 1: Overhead Squat and Snatch Pull Combination

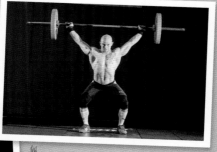

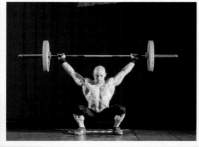

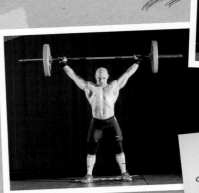

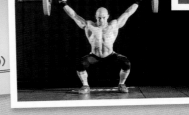

10 overhead squats (page 100)

Combined with

10 snatch pulls from the floor (page 60)

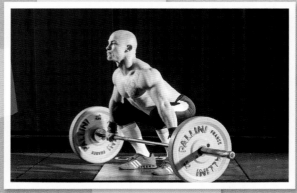

Do three circuits of this combination, taking 30 sec to 1 min of rest.

②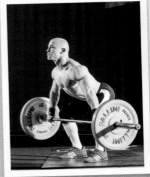

③

④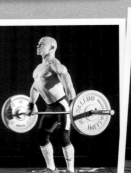

⑤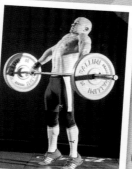

Exercise 2: Snatch Pulls From the Midthigh and Hang Clean Combination

10 snatch pulls from the midthigh (page 60)

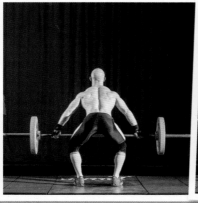

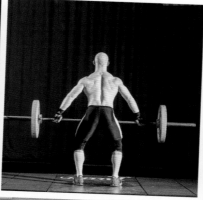

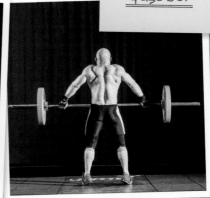

①

②

+

10 hang cleans (page 34)

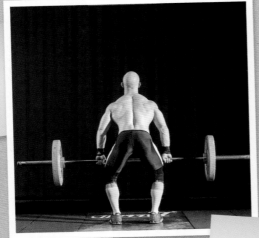

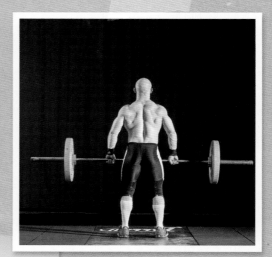

Repeat this combination three times, taking 30 sec to 1 min of rest.

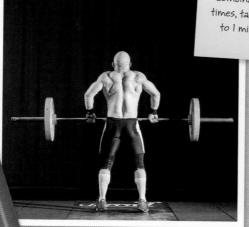

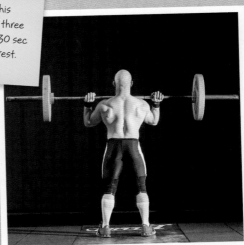

③

④

Exercise 3:
Clean and Jerk Combination

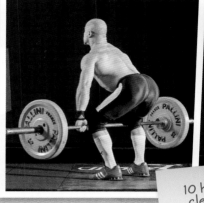

①

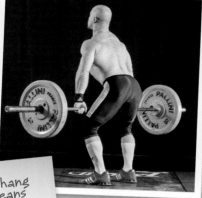

②

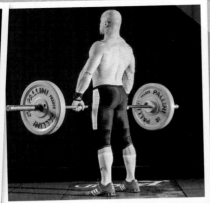

③

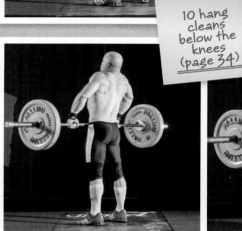

④

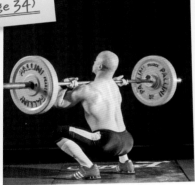

⑤

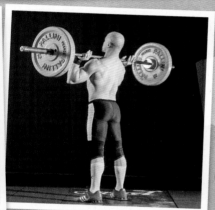

⑥

10 hang cleans below the knees (page 34)

Combine with

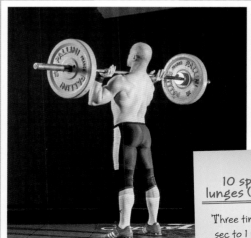

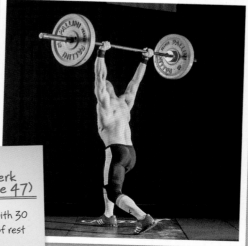

10 split jerk lunges (page 47)

Three times with 30 sec to 1 min of rest

Finish with two to three sets of three clean and jerks with 1 to 2 min of rest between sets.

Light Kettlebell Routine (with no rest)

Do this combination without any rest breaks. Repeat two to three times, taking 30 sec to 1 min of rest between rounds.

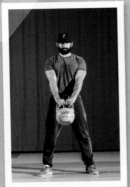
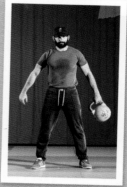
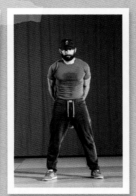
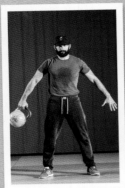
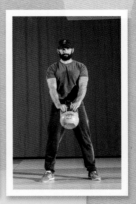

20 rotations around the waist (10 on each side)

Combined with

10 forward alternating lunges

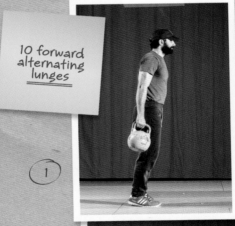

①

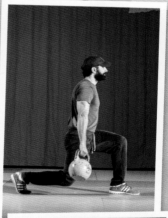

②

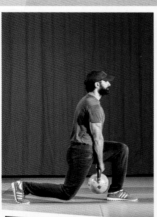

③

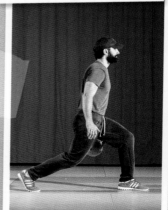

④

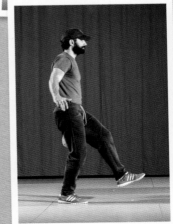

⑤

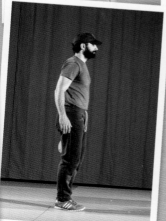

⑥

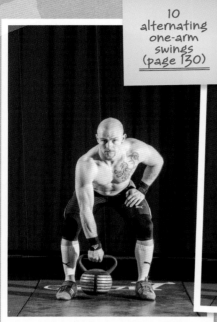

10 alternating one-arm swings (page 130)

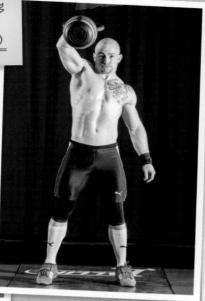

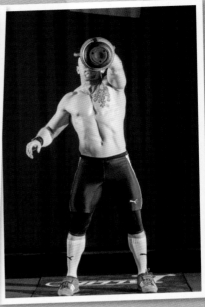

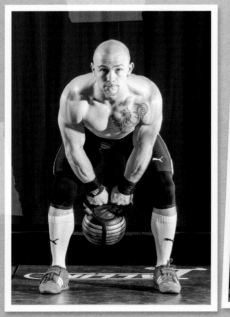

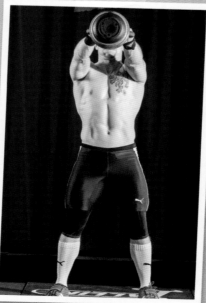

Russian variation

10 two-arm kettlebell swings (page 129)

See the American variation on the next page.

American variation

See the Russian variation on the previous page.

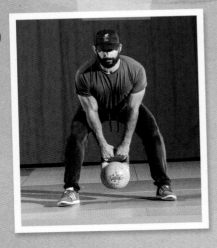

(1)

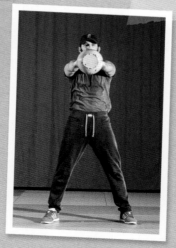

(2)

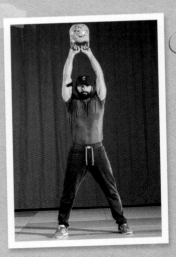

(3)

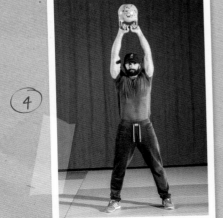

(4)

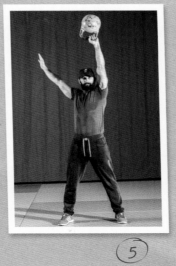

(5)

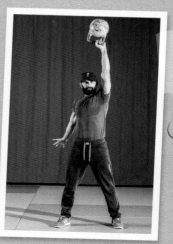

(6)

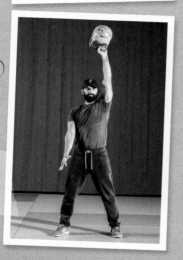

(7)

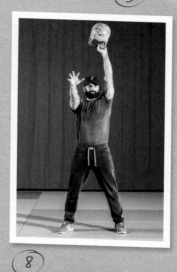

(8)

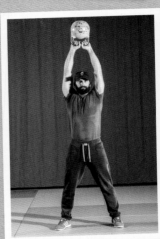

(9)

10 kettlebell swings and 180-degree turn

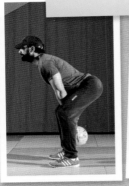

(1)

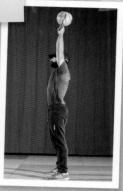

(2)

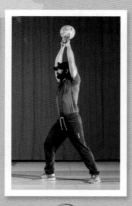

(3)

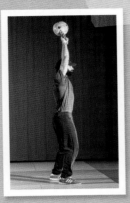

(4)

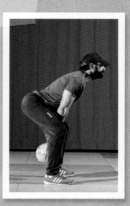

(5)

Sandbag Routine

Do the exercises one after the other. You may rest for a few seconds after each exercise. Do two to three sets, taking 30 sec to 1 min of rest.

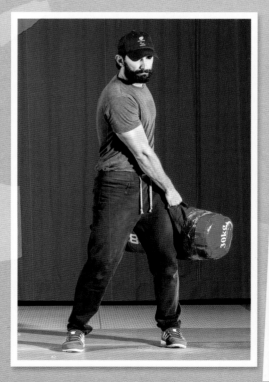

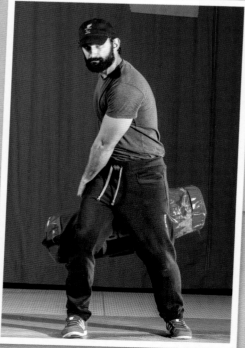

10 torso rotations

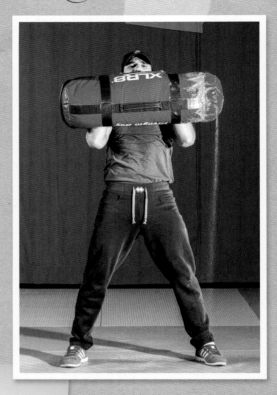

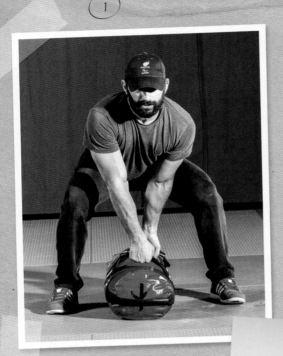

10 deadlifts
with overhead
press

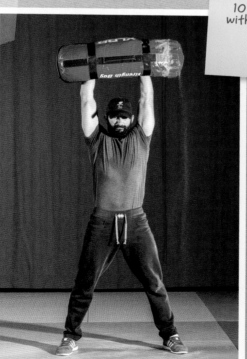

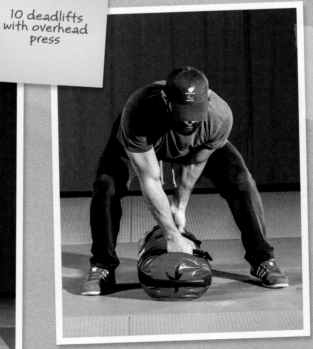

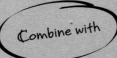

Combine with

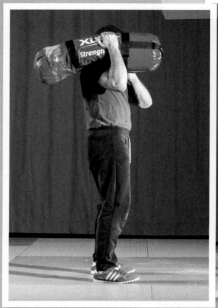

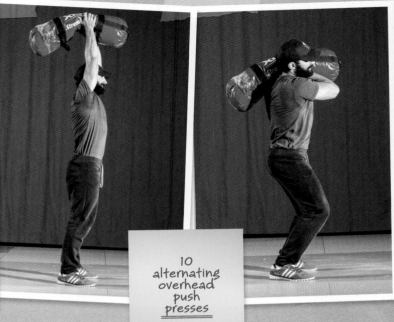

10
alternating
overhead
push
presses

Then

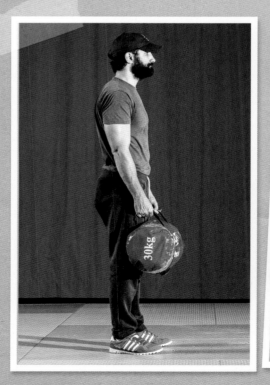

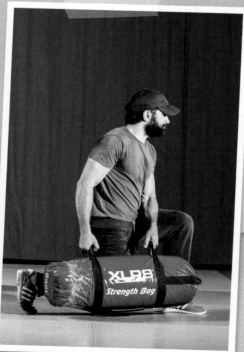

10 lunges with
side rotation

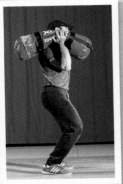
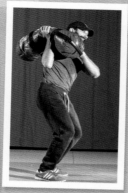
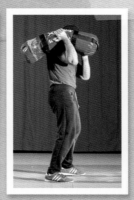
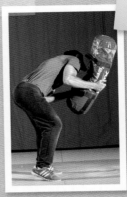
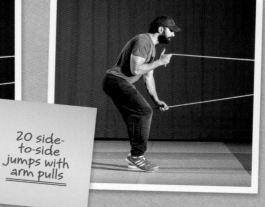

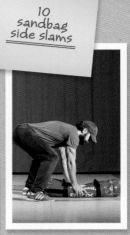

10 sandbag side slams

Band Routine

Combine these exercises with no breaks. Do two to three sets, with 30 sec to 1 min of rest between sets.

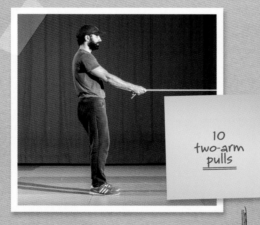
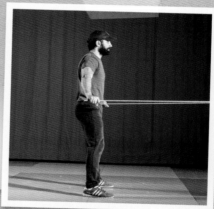

10 two-arm pulls

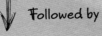
Followed by

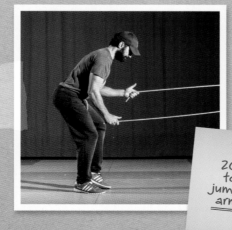

20 side-to-side jumps with arm pulls

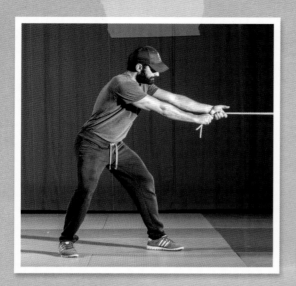

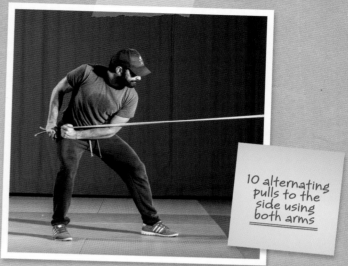

10 alternating
pulls to the
side using
both arms

Then

① ② ③

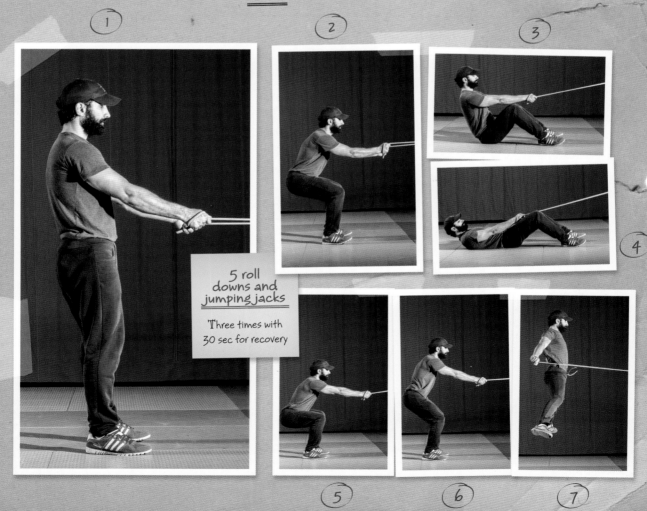

5 roll
downs and
jumping jacks

Three times with
30 sec for recovery

④

⑤ ⑥ ⑦

Landmine Routine With a Bar

Do the following four exercises without breaking your rhythm. Use a comfortable weight so that you can focus on your technique. Do three sets with 30 sec to 1 min for recovery.

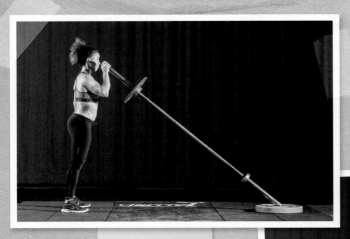

10 squats

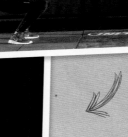

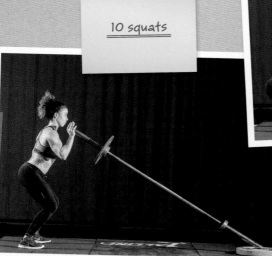

10 bar pushes with alternating hands

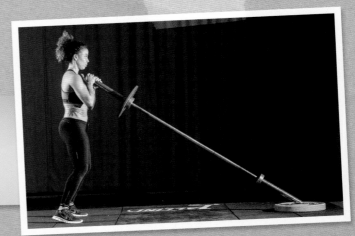

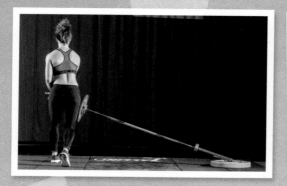

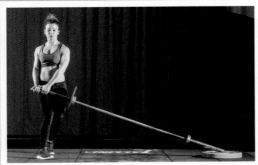

10 oblique twists

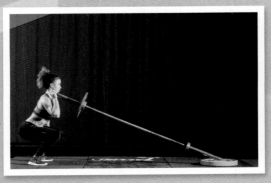

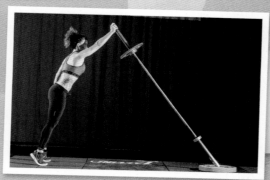

10 thrusters

Battle Rope Routine

Do the following exercises and take 10 sec to recover after each exercise. You may repeat the entire circuit after 1 min of rest.

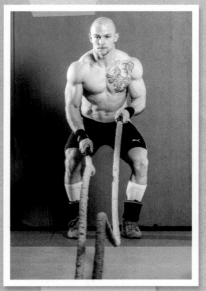

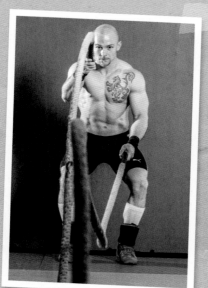

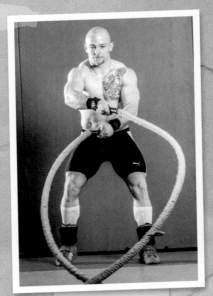

10 normal waves (page 176)

10 sec of recovery while jumping

10 large waves (page 176)

10 sec of recovery while jumping

10 crossing waves (page 177)

10 sec of recovery while jumping

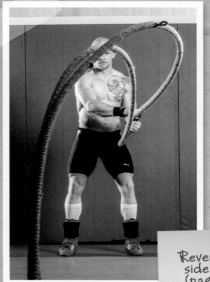

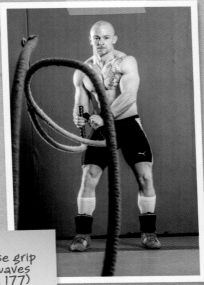

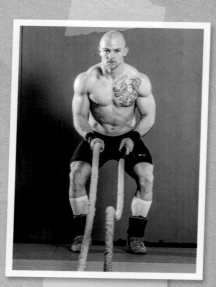

Reverse grip
side waves
(page 177)

10 sec of recovery
while jumping

Short
and rapid
waves for 20
to 30 sec

One to two rounds
with 1 min of recovery

Suspension Strap Routine

Exercise 1: ITW

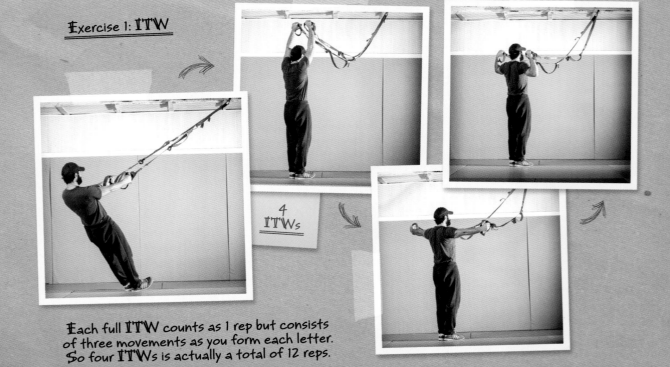

4
ITWs

Each full ITW counts as 1 rep but consists
of three movements as you form each letter.
So four ITWs is actually a total of 12 reps.

Exercise 2: Pistol Squats

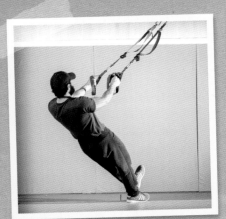
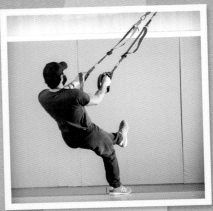
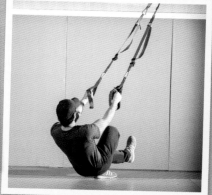

10 pistol squats
per leg x 3

Exercise 3: Superman

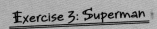

① ②

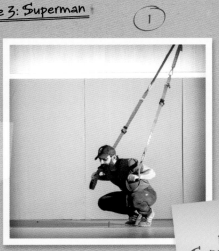
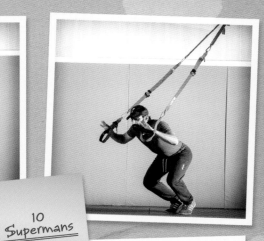

10
Supermans

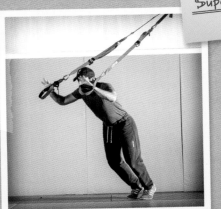
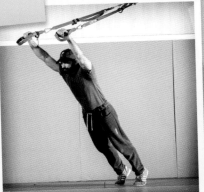

③ ④

Exercise 4: Push-Ups

10 push-ups
x 3

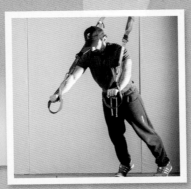
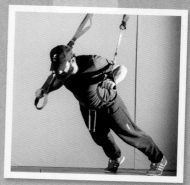

Exercise 5: Suspended Knee Tucks

10 suspended knee tucks

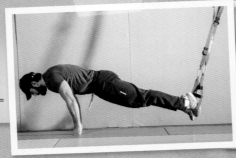
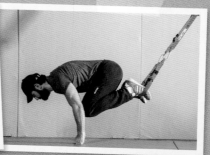

Finish with

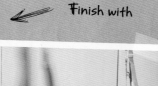

Exercise 6: Leg Curls

10 leg curls
x 3

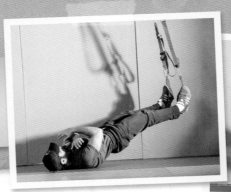

Athletic Routine

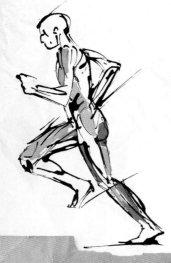

Perform this routine two to three times with 1 min of recovery:
100 m run at a moderate pace, 25 m with high knees, 25 m butt kick, 25 m with right high knee only, 25 m with left high knee only, 25 m butt kick (right side only), 25 m butt kick (left side only), 25 m skip, 25 m run with straight legs, 100 m run at a moderate pace.

Chapter 2

TECHNICAL FOUNDATION

034   Foundational Exercises

034   Clean and Jerk

089   Basic Athletic Exercises

089   Squat
120   Bench Press
125   Deadlift

143   Bodyweight Exercises

143   Foundation for Pull-Ups
158   Push-Up
169   Explosive Push-Up
174   Battle Ropes
180   Dips
182   Core Exercises

192   Running

194   Parameters of Running
195   Mechanics of Stride Adaptation

FOUNDATIONAL EXERCISES

Weightlifting exercises play an enormous role in high intensity training (and in resistance training in general). The technical skills required make these exercises the movements of choice for anyone who wants to make rapid progress without spending long hours training. Although the basic exercises have many versions—semitechnical and educational exercises that simplify the movements so that they can be mastered or so that heavier weights can be used—we will start with two classic exercises from Olympic competitions: the clean and jerk and the snatch.

✖ CLEAN AND JERK

This exercise is slightly less technical than the snatch, and it requires a bit more power and strength. It is made up of two distinct movements: the clean and the jerk.

CLEAN

This movement has six successive and distinct parts.

➲ Part 1—Starting position

The starting position is close to the bar with the shoulders, knees, and toes facing forward. The shoulders are slightly in front of the knees, and the knees are slightly in front of the front of the feet. The feet are planted firmly, flat on the floor.

The width of the feet can vary from one person to another, but the general recommendation is to begin with the feet a bit wider than hip-width apart, because the stance will widen as the bar is raised.

Grab the bar using an overhand grip with the hands about shoulder-width apart. Lastly, with the back in a natural lumbar curve, squeeze your shoulder blades together and hold them in this position.

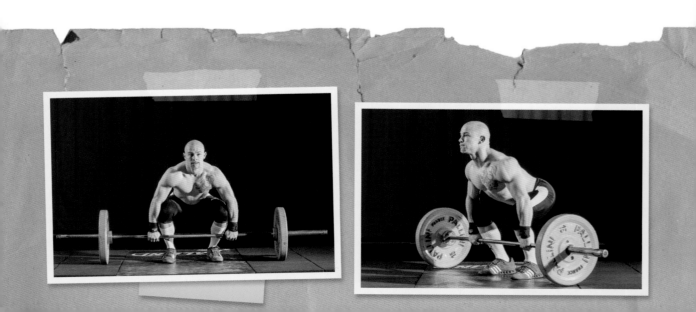

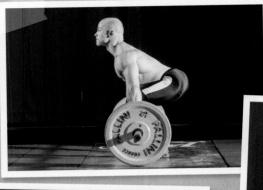

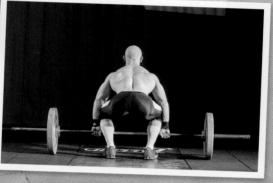

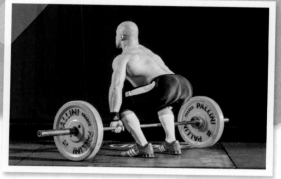

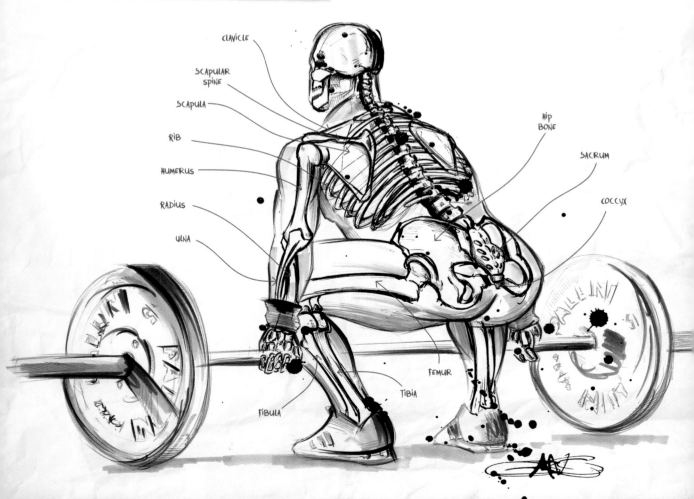

CLAVICLE

SCAPULAR SPINE

SCAPULA

RIB

HUMERUS

RADIUS

ULNA

HIP BONE

SACRUM

COCCYX

FEMUR

TIBIA

FIBULA

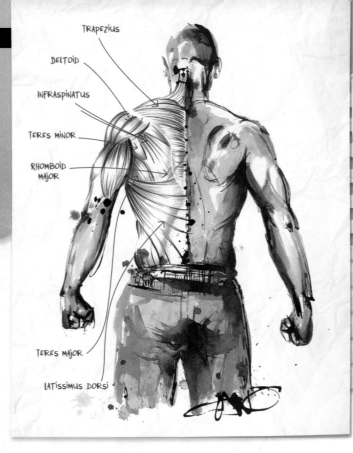

TRAPEZIUS
DELTOID
INFRASPINATUS
TERES MINOR
RHOMBOID MAJOR
TERES MAJOR
LATISSIMUS DORSI

Squeeze the shoulder blades together

Most of the everyday back pain that people experience is the result of an overpronounced kyphosis (curvature of the spine) with the shoulders rounded forward. This posture often happens because of weak muscles in the rotator cuff and surrounding the shoulder blades.

If you are having trouble correcting this posture, you must strengthen these muscles. During your workout, you can activate them by sticking out your chest, pulling your shoulders back, and squeezing the shoulder blades together. This position will limit the kyphosis, flatten the back, strengthen it, and protect it, all while making it more powerful.

Part 2—The first pull

This part is the first time the bar moves, coming from the floor to the knees. Initiated by the knees, the second part is done with straight arms and without changing the angle of the back. Then, to allow the bar to pass by the knees, the knees move backward slightly and bend a little, moving the bar from the floor to just above the knee. During this part, your weight will shift to the balls of your feet but your heels will still be on the floor. The quadriceps, glutes, and hamstrings are recruited during the first pull, stabilized by the spinal, back, and paravertebral muscles.

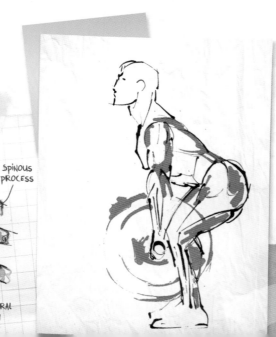

DISC
SPINOUS PROCESS
VERTEBRAL BODY

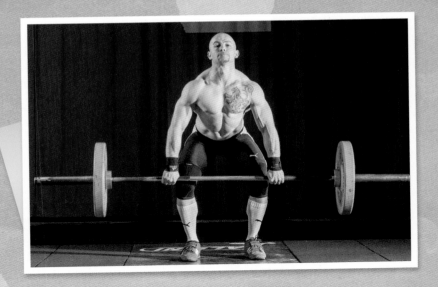

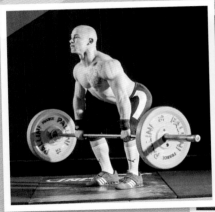

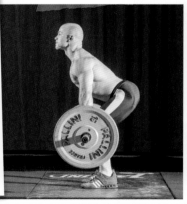

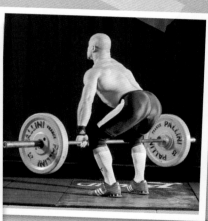

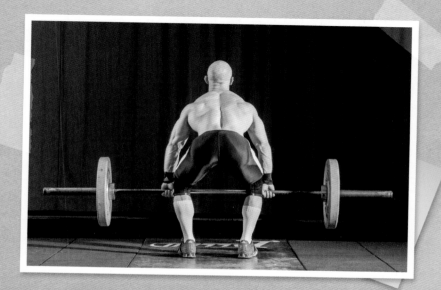

➲ Part 3—Transition

In this part, the movement slows down; therefore, it should be as brief as possible. This part is preparing you for the second critical acceleration that happens in part 4. During this transition, the back straightens slightly to allow the knees to reengage under the bar, and the bar slides up to midthigh. The feet remain flat on the floor as the weight shifts from the toes to the heels and finally to the soles of the feet.

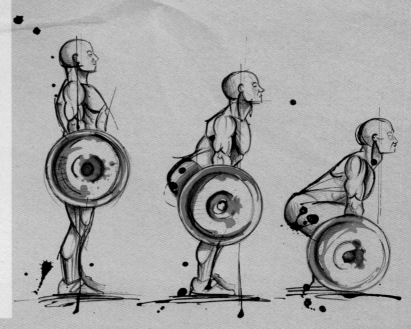

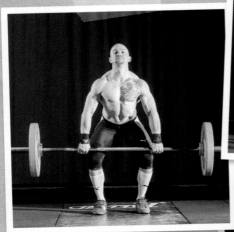

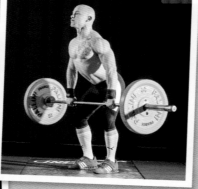

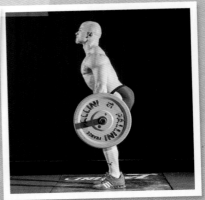

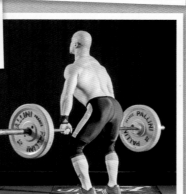

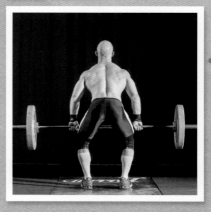

Part 4—The second pull

Just like the first pull, this part is driven by a large push from the legs that drives the bar upward and helps the arms pull (lifting the shoulders and then the elbows) before they go under the bar. The front part of the feet lift up as the back straightens, driving the pelvis forward.

A large number of muscles are used in this part; practically the entire body is working to support the large muscle groups.

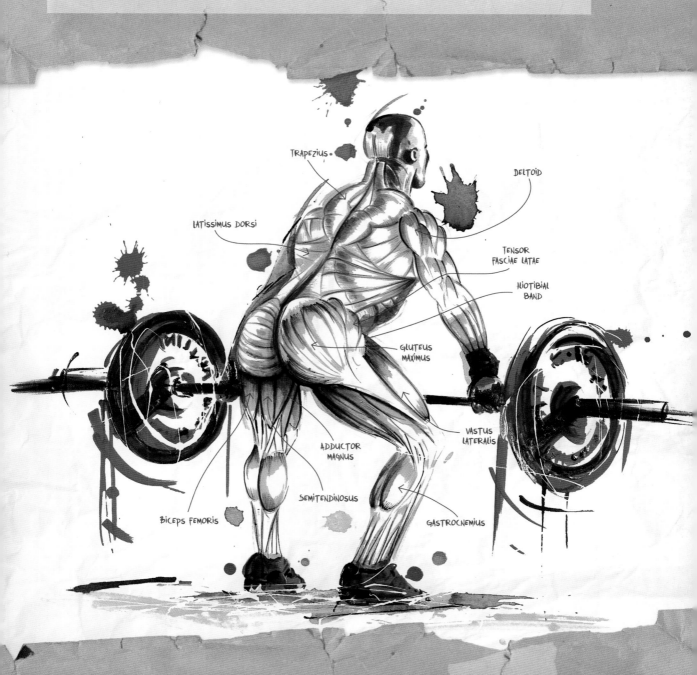

TRAPEZIUS

DELTOID

LATISSIMUS DORSI

TENSOR FASCIAE LATAE

ILIOTIBIAL BAND

GLUTEUS MAXIMUS

VASTUS LATERALIS

ADDUCTOR MAGNUS

SEMITENDINOSUS

BICEPS FEMORIS

GASTROCNEMIUS

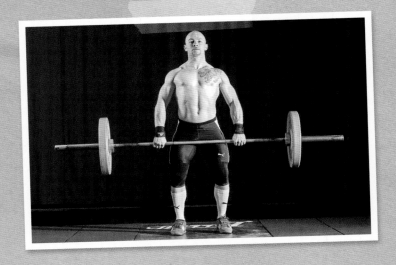

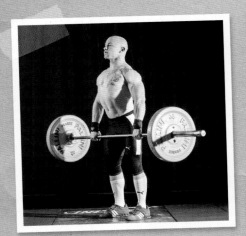

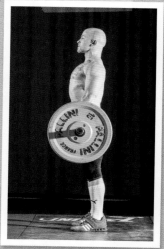

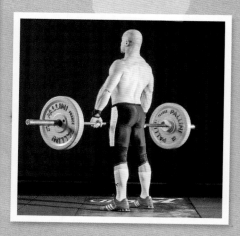

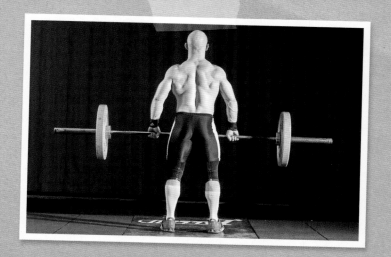

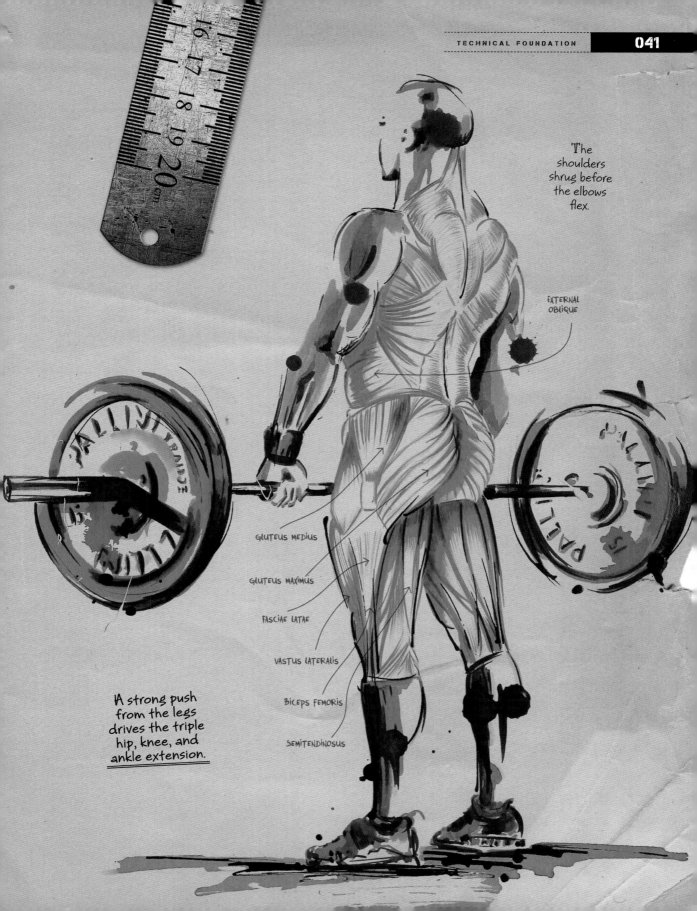

The shoulders shrug before the elbows flex.

EXTERNAL OBLIQUE

GLUTEUS MEDIUS

GLUTEUS MAXIMUS

FASCIAE LATAE

VASTUS LATERALIS

BICEPS FEMORIS

SEMITENDINOSUS

A strong push from the legs drives the triple hip, knee, and ankle extension.

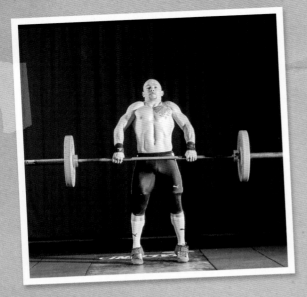

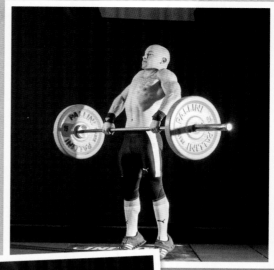

The mechanics of ankle extension (plantar flexion)

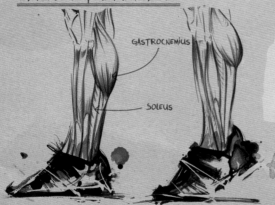

GASTROCNEMIUS

SOLEUS

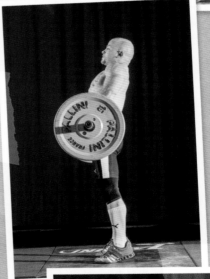

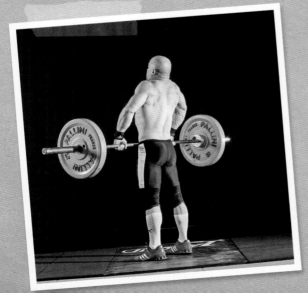

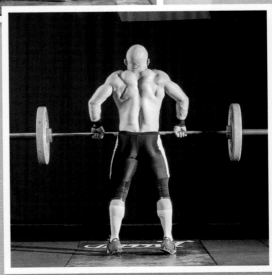

➲ Part 5—Sliding under the bar

Using the momentum generated during the second pull, the trapezius, shoulders, and arm muscles lift the bar higher, allowing you to slide under it so that you end up with your elbows to the front and the bar touching your clavicles. During the jump to move under the bar, move your feet out to the sides for increased stability.

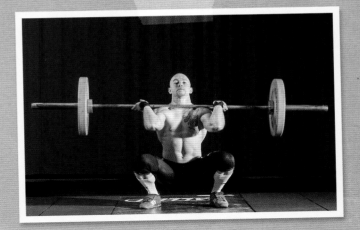

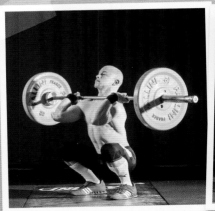
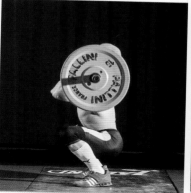
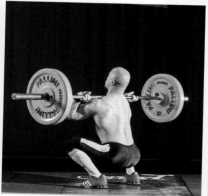

The pelvis is held stable primarily by the abdominal muscles, the spinal muscles, and the hamstrings.

The abdominal and spinal muscles also actively support the torso. The shoulders, arms, back, and paravertebral muscles support the upper back and shoulder blades.

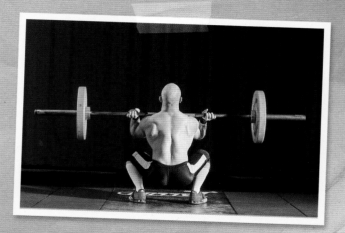

⊙ Part 6—Standing back up

After your feet hit the floor, fully stand up using a concentric action of the quadriceps and glutes. At the end of the movement, the feet return to their normal position, the pelvis is tilted slightly forward, the chest is open wide, the elbows are forward, and the torso is strongly supported.

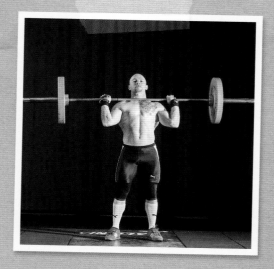

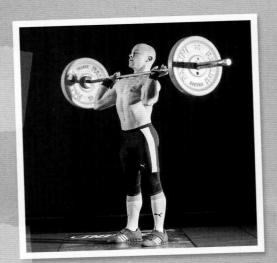

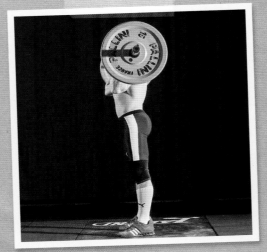

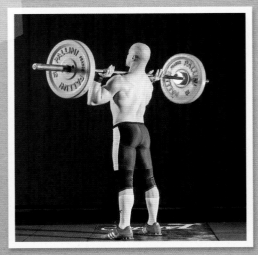

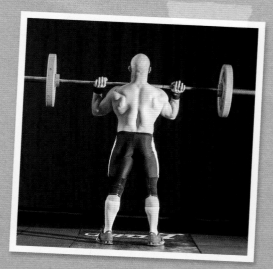

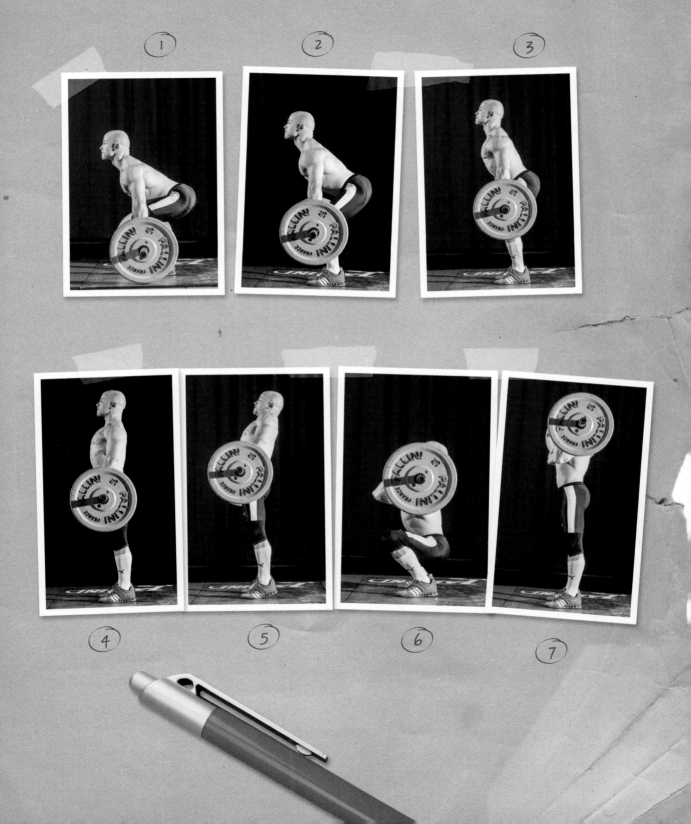

WORKOUT - CLEANS

WORKOUT 1 - NORDIC COMBINATIONS

12 SETS, EVERY MINUTE, ALTERNATING:

EVEN SETS: 2 CLEANS, 2 HANG CLEANS, 2 ALTERNATING
SPLIT JERK LUNGES (PAGE 47)

ODD SETS: 4 WEIGHTED DIPS (PAGE 80)

RECOVERY: 4 MINUTES OF RUNNING

21, 15, 9 REPS OF BAR SQUATS (PAGE 89) AS FAST AS POSSIBLE
ALTERNATED WITH BURPEES (PAGE 165) AND THEN BOX JUMPS

WORKOUT 2 - ENGLISH BREAKFAST

3 X 10 FRONT SQUATS (PAGE 97)

3 X 10 FULL PULL-UPS WITH BANDS (PAGE 143)

3 X 3 DEADLIFTS (PAGE 125), 1 CLEAN,
3 FRONT SQUATS (PAGE 97), 1 JERK (PAGE 47)

RECOVER FOR 90 SECONDS, REPEAT 5 TIMES.

WORKOUT 3 - PUSH-UPS TO SQUATS NOT CLEAN

REPEAT AS MANY TIMES AS POSSIBLE IN 3 MINUTES:
3 CLEANS, 6 PUSH-UPS (PAGE 158), 9 SQUATS (PAGE 95)

REPEAT THIS COMBINATION FIVE TIMES, TAKING 1
MINUTE OF REST AFTER EACH ROUND.

JERK

The second part of the clean and jerk can be divided into four parts.

⊙ Part 1—The dip

At the end of the clean, the bar is touching the clavicles. The chest is open, and the elbows are lifted very high in front. Keep your head straight and your gaze fixed on a point just above the horizon. Your feet are now in the original starting position, about hip-width apart. A quarter squat, done with control, provides enough momentum to start the movement. The feet should be flat on the floor with the weight on the soles. Throughout the movement, you must maintain your form to support the upper back and torso. The hamstrings play an essential part in halting the descent and stabilizing the pelvis

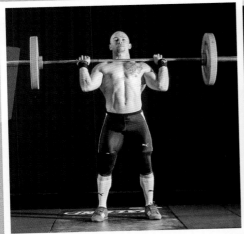
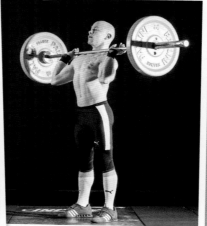
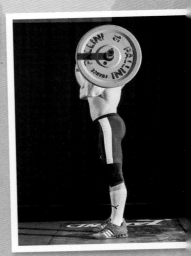
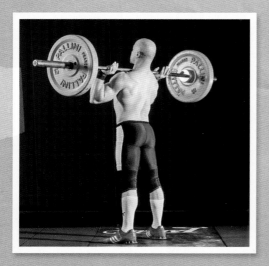
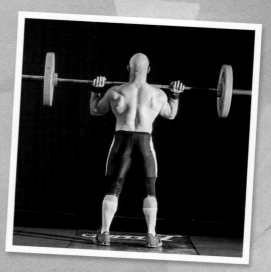

➲ Part 2—The drive

Using the rebound momentum from the dip, a combined push from the quadriceps, glutes, and calves is transferred by the action of the deltoids and trapezius muscles into a shoulder shrug. The arms should stay in position and relaxed throughout this dynamic vertical extension of the lower limbs so as not to interfere with the drive upward. At the end of the drive, height is important; from the shoulders to the ankles, the joints must be in alignment. The head moves slightly backward so that the bar does not hit the chin as it leaves the shoulders.

➲ Part 3—Passage

The drive, along with a jump, allows you to go under the bar. By pushing the bar as you jump, you actually push your body down toward the ground so that you end up in a lunge position with arms straight overhead. This new position requires total core support to balance the bar and your body and involves a concentric contraction of the triceps and deltoids with an isometric hold. The bar is balanced just behind the head. The forward foot pushes into the floor for stability. The front and back thighs should form angles greater than 90 degrees. Be careful not to rotate your back leg outward, because doing so will rotate your foot outward as well. Also, you need to keep the pelvis tilted forward.

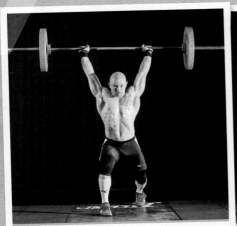
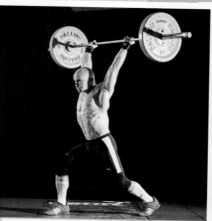
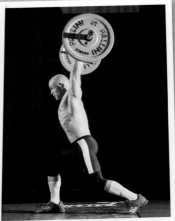
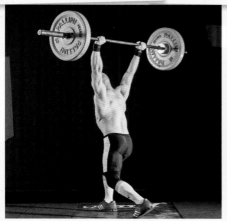
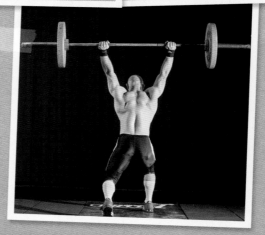

➔ Part 4—Return

Return to standing position by first pulling your front foot back and then bringing your back foot forward. Then you can drop the bar to the ground.

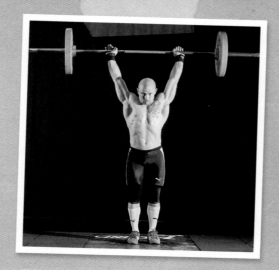

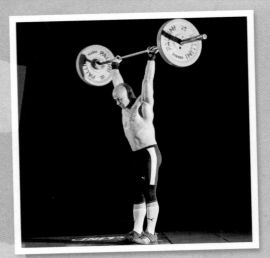

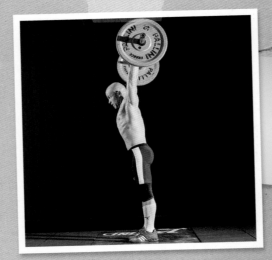

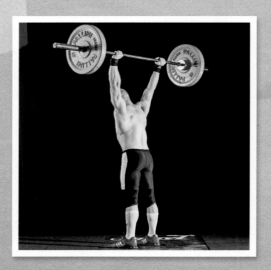

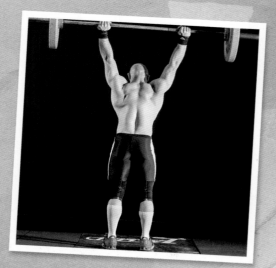

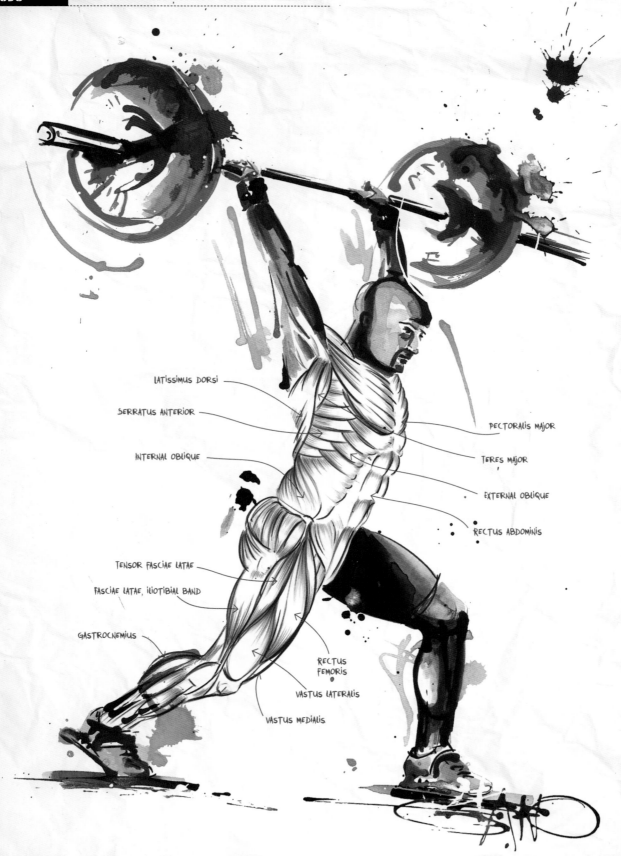

LATISSIMUS DORSI

SERRATUS ANTERIOR

INTERNAL OBLIQUE

PECTORALIS MAJOR

TERES MAJOR

EXTERNAL OBLIQUE

RECTUS ABDOMINIS

TENSOR FASCIAE LATAE

FASCIAE LATAE, ILIOTIBIAL BAND

GASTROCNEMIUS

RECTUS FEMORIS

VASTUS LATERALIS

VASTUS MEDIALIS

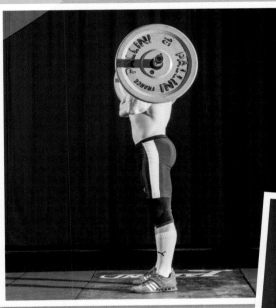

Flex your legs slightly, and . . .

jump!

The front leg comes
back and then

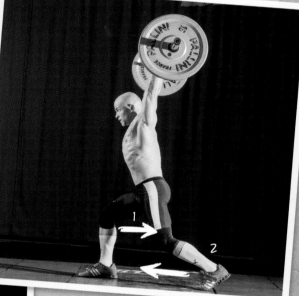

the back leg moves forward.
The lunge must be deep enough.

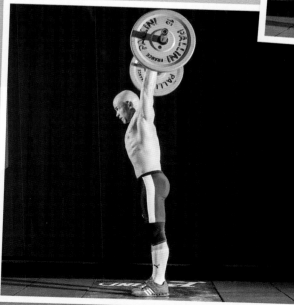

WORKOUT — JERKS

WORKOUT 1 — REVERSE RUN

DO AS MANY ROUNDS AS
POSSIBLE IN 12 MINUTES:

15 BOX JUMPS, 15 JERKS (PAGE 47),
300-METER REVERSE RUN

WORKOUT 2 — IT'S EXPLOSIVE, BUT IT WON'T HURT

DO EVERY MINUTE FOR 20 MINUTES:

50-METER SPRINT, 4 JERKS (PAGE 47),
6 BURPEES (PAGE 165)

WORKOUT 3 — DISCOVER THE TRUTH

YOU HAVE 17 MINUTES TO FIND YOUR MAXIMUM IN THE DEADLIFT
(PAGE 125), SQUAT (PAGE 89), AND JERK (PAGE 47). HOW YOU
MANAGE THE TIME AND THE EXERCISES IS UP TO YOU. OF
COURSE, YOU NEED TO REACH THE HIGHEST WEIGHT POSSIBLE.

Why reverse running?

Obviously, you run more slowly backward than you do forward. Running slower is not a problem in workouts when you are repeating below maximum intensity exercises, not high intensity ones. Reverse running is an effective and original exercise that develops the posterior chain in a functional and surprising way. In this exercise, you always strike the ground with the front of the foot first, which limits the impact, develops proprioceptive qualities in the foot, and improves your running technique.

WORKOUT - CLEAN AND JERKS

WORKOUT 1 - TO INFINITY

DO 1 CLEAN AND JERK (PAGES 34, 47), 1 SQUAT (PAGE 89), AND 1 BARBELL AB ROLLOUT ON THE KNEES (PAGE 190). ADD 2 REPS TO THE LAST TWO EXERCISES WITH EVERY ROUND. SO, YOU DO

1 CLEAN AND JERK, 3 SQUATS, 3 BARBELL AB ROLLOUTS,
1 CLEAN AND JERK, 5 SQUATS, 5 BARBELL AB ROLLOUTS,
AND SO ON.

YOU HAVE NO TIME LIMIT, BUT YOU SHOULD DO AS MANY REPS AS POSSIBLE. IF YOU STOP DURING A SET, THE REP COUNT STOPS.

WORKOUT 2 - TECHNICAL DEVELOPMENT

4 X 5 FRONT SQUATS (PAGE 97)

4 X 3 CLEAN AND JERKS (PAGES 34, 47)

4 X 3 HANG CLEANS

3 X CLEAN, FRONT SQUAT, JERK EVERY MINUTE FOR 7 MINUTES

WORKOUT 3 - NITRO

DO 15 SETS WITH 2 MINUTES OF RECOVERY BETWEEN ROUNDS:

3 CLEANS (PAGE 34), 6 BOX JUMPS, 30-METER SPRINT

SANDBAG CLEAN

This variation uses a sandbag instead of a weight bar. Still, because the weight is lighter and the sandbag is harder to control than a bar, your form can quickly be compromised. Be careful to keep the sandbag close to your body throughout the exercise (do not let it fall forward).

Whether you are lifting the sandbag from the floor or from above the knees, it is important to use the triple hip, knee, and ankle extension to lift the sandbag as high as you can while keeping it close to your body. The sandbag clean is divided into a shoulder shrug and then a rotation of the sandbag toward the body so that it ends up resting on the arms. The sandbag should be received in a quarter or half squat with the back straight and the head lifted.

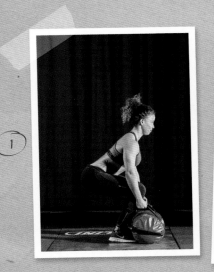

1

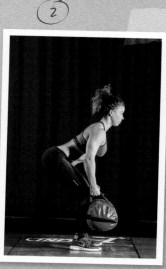

2

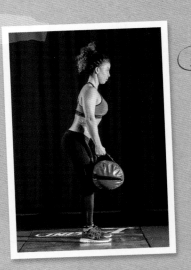

3

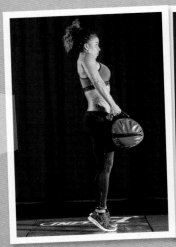

4

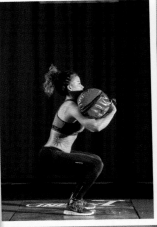

5

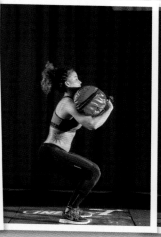

6

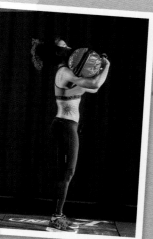

7

WORKOUT - SANDBAGS

WORKOUT 1 - RANDOM TIME CIRCUIT

TASK 1: SANDBAG CLEANS
TASK 2: BURPEES (PAGE 165) ON THE BAG
TASK 3: PASS THE BAG FROM ONE SHOULDER TO THE OTHER
TASK 4: SIDE JUMPS OVER THE BAG
TASK 5: LIFT THE BAG, PUT IT ON YOUR SHOULDER, THROW IT
ON THE GROUND (SWITCH SHOULDERS FOR EACH REP)
DO THE TASKS IN ORDER FOR 17 MINUTES; YOU CAN SPEND
HOWEVER MUCH TIME YOU NEED FOR EACH ONE.

WORKOUT 2 - CONTAMINATED SANDBAG

EVERY MINUTE FOR 10 MINUTES:

5 CLEANS (PAGE 34), 5 BURPEES ON THE BAG (PAGE 165),
5 FRONT SQUATS (PAGE 97), 5 KNEE TUCK JUMPS ABOVE THE BAG

RECOVERY: 3 MINUTES OF LOW INTENSITY JOGGING

AS MANY TIMES AS YOU CAN IN 6 MINUTES:

2 CLEANS, PUT THE BAG ON ONE SHOULDER,
THROW IT ON THE GROUND; 30-METER SPRINT;
6 BURPEES, 30-METER SPRINT;
2 CLEANS; PUT THE BAG ON ONE SHOULDER,
THROW IT ON THE GROUND; AND SO ON.

WORKOUT 3 - EXPLOSIVE SANDBAG

10 ROUNDS: SANDBAG CLEAN, SANDBAG
SQUAT, THROW THE BAG AS FAR AS YOU
CAN, MAXIMUM VERTICAL JUMP, 30-METER
SPRINT. RECOVERY FOR 2 MINUTES.

Forget long sets

Because you are reading this book, you probably understand why people love the many variations of high intensity training. But do you know why it comes under scrutiny? Because injuries can occur. They can happen during long sets of many reps of technical exercises such as clean and jerks or snatches. Also, remember that long sets may be ineffective as we discussed earlier in this book (see the section on training interference). In addition, the complex movement patterns and the cognitive demand of cleans or snatches combined with the high levels of lactate produced by long sets negatively affect muscle contraction efficacy and strength and power output.

TIRE CLEAN

By now, you understand the importance of proper technique for exercises that are commonly used in high intensity training. Despite how often versions of the clean and jerk or snatch are used in a workout, we should not forget the virtue of including a wild, fun variation such as the tire flip. This exercise is just a clean and jerk with a tire.

Sometimes, athletes may start a workout or do an exercise without proper control over the back. The result is that they end up doing an exercise such as the tire flip with a rounded back, sometimes for several dozen reps. If the lack of vertebral support is not caused by current low back pain (see the box about vertebral pathologies on page 58), then the fun part of the workout takes over and they cease to pay attention to having correct back position. But a tire flip can be done safely. First, use lightweight tires. Doing several reps with control is better than giving a demonstration of absolute strength consisting of one flip with a rounded back.

Because the tire is on the ground, you need to spread your legs wider apart and flex your hips and knees more than you do for the clean and jerk.

◉ Technique tips

The movement begins with a deep bend in the legs and the hips wide open to protect the knees from the tire during the upward movement. Thus, hip and ankle flexibility are important here. Keep your arms straight and slide your fingers underneath the tire.

Before applying any tension, lower your buttocks as much as you can to get as close to the floor as possible. The back should be as flat as possible (if you cannot flatten your back, then we advise against doing this exercise).

Your weight should be slightly toward your heels, but it will quickly move toward the balls of your feet.

With your chest open and your chin lifted so that it does not hit the tire, squeeze your shoulder blades together and begin the first pull. During the first pull, you must lift the tire as high as you can and as quickly as you can so that you can slide under it in the clean position. To do this, use your lower limbs to push hard against the floor as you stand up and press your hips forward. Your weight will move toward the front, up to the balls of your feet.

Your feet return to being flat on the floor (in the case of a lunge, only the front foot should be flat) as you receive the tire. You can receive the tire in a one-third squat or a partial lunge. In a lunge position, you should keep your legs and feet parallel.

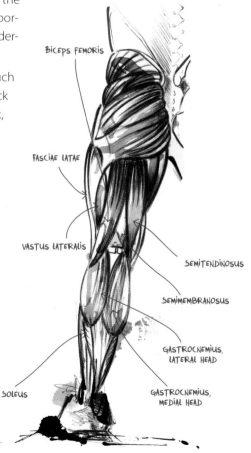

BICEPS FEMORIS

FASCIAE LATAE

VASTUS LATERALIS

SEMITENDINOSUS

SEMIMEMBRANOSUS

GASTROCNEMIUS, LATERAL HEAD

SOLEUS

GASTROCNEMIUS, MEDIAL HEAD

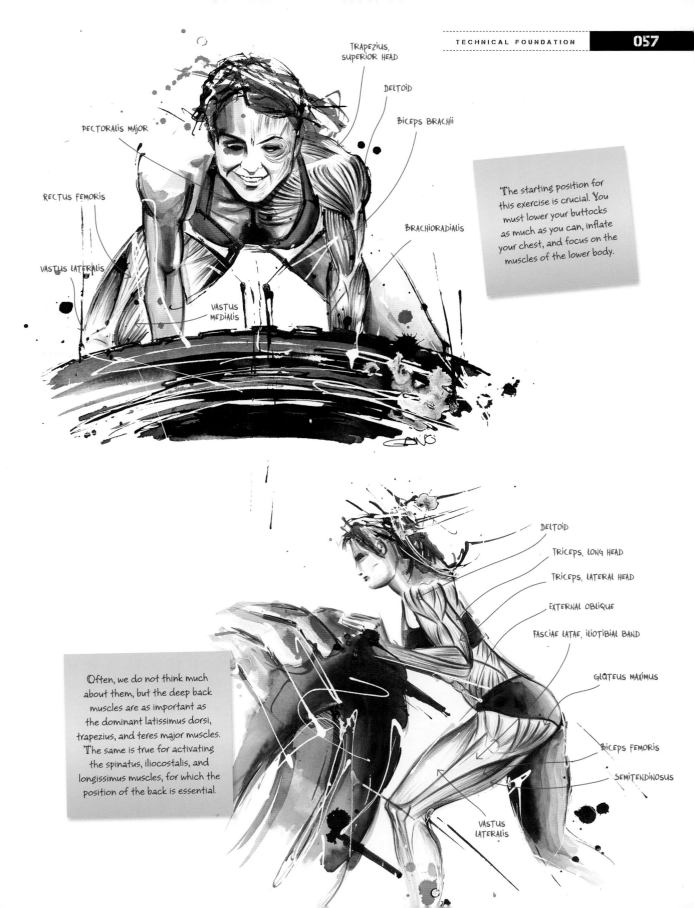

TRAPEZIUS, SUPERIOR HEAD

DELTOID

BICEPS BRACHII

PECTORALIS MAJOR

BRACHIORADIALIS

RECTUS FEMORIS

VASTUS LATERALIS

VASTUS MEDIALIS

The starting position for this exercise is crucial. You must lower your buttocks as much as you can, inflate your chest, and focus on the muscles of the lower body.

DELTOID

TRICEPS, LONG HEAD

TRICEPS, LATERAL HEAD

EXTERNAL OBLIQUE

FASCIAE LATAE, ILIOTIBIAL BAND

GLUTEUS MAXIMUS

BICEPS FEMORIS

SEMITENDINOSUS

VASTUS LATERALIS

Often, we do not think much about them, but the deep back muscles are as important as the dominant latissimus dorsi, trapezius, and teres major muscles. The same is true for activating the spinatus, iliocostalis, and longissimus muscles, for which the position of the back is essential.

Herniated disc

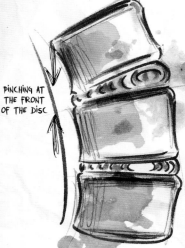

MATERIAL IS PUSHED OUT.

PINCHING AT
THE FRONT
OF THE DISC

The threat to your discs

Those people who place themselves in the best position to lift a weight are those who currently have, or who have had, back pain. Indeed, when you are in pain, you have no other choice: You must always control the forward tilt of the pelvis, keep your back flat, keep the vertebrae aligned, and support the muscles that surround and protect the spine.

To avoid problems, you must be obsessive about the position of your back and be serious about technique when doing squats, deadlifts, cleans, snatches, and upright rows.

The main danger is a herniated disc. Intervertebral discs are cushions between all the vertebrae; they absorb shock and provide stability and mobility in the spine. The center of each disc contains a "gel." When the back is curved forward (rounded), the gel is pushed backward as the front of the disc is pinched and the back opens up. If the pressure in the front increases, especially under a heavy distal weight, the gel could be pushed outside the disc. The result is a herniated disc.

Repetitive movements done with the spine in an incorrect position can also cause local muscle inflammation, damage the discs (making them age prematurely), cause arthritis, and so on.

Bad form

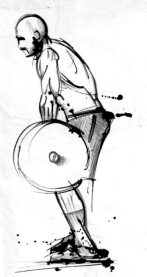

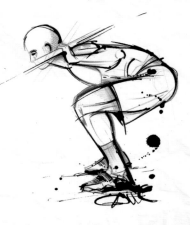

WORKOUT - TIRE CLEANS

WORKOUT 1 - TIRED

REPEAT THE FOLLOWING CIRCUIT 3 TIMES AS QUICKLY AS POSSIBLE:

8 TIRE FLIPS, 20 TIRE JUMPS, 15 BURPEES (PAGE 165), 400-METER RUN

WORKOUT 2 - MARIO

10, 9, 8, 7, 6, 5, 4, 3, 2, 1 THRUSTERS (PAGE 103).
EACH SET IS FOLLOWED BY A TIRE FLIP.

90 SECONDS OF RECOVERY BETWEEN SETS

WORKOUT 3 - WEIGHTLIFTER SPRINT

DO 10 SETS WITH 3 TO 4 MINUTES OF REST:

1 CLEAN AND JERK (PAGES 34, 47), 1 TIRE FLIP, 60-METER SPRINT

SNATCH

Eminently technical, this exercise has turned off more than one athlete. But if you take the time to learn it, it will give you maximum return on your investment. As with the clean and jerk, we can break this exercise into five parts.

- -

➲ Part 1—Starting position

Use an overhand (pronated) grip on the bar with your hands wider than shoulder-width apart. The shoulders, knees, and toes are in front of the bar, and the bar is touching the shins. The shoulders should be just in front of the knees, the knees just in front of the toes, and the arms straight. The feet are flat on the floor with the weight on the soles. Your feet should be about hip-width apart and slightly turned out. Finally, with the back in a natural lumbar curve, squeeze your shoulder blades together and hold them in this position.

Wide grip

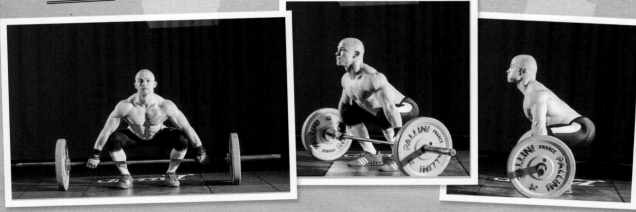

The feet are flat on the floor with the weight on the soles of the feet.

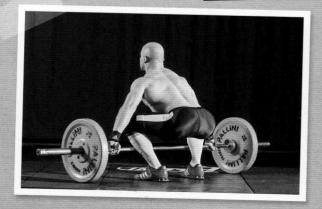

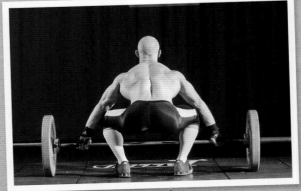

The back is in alignment in a natural lumbar curve.

➲ Part 2—The first pull

Just as in the clean, this is the first time you move the bar, going from the floor to the knees. The arms are straight during the first pull, and the back stays in position. The drive comes from the lower limbs, and the knees move slightly as you lift the bar off the floor to just past the kneecaps. But the legs remain flexed. Your weight shifts to the balls of your feet.

This part of the exercise recruits the quadriceps, glutes, hamstrings, and the spinal, back, and paravertebral muscles provide stability.

The speed of the first pull is essential.

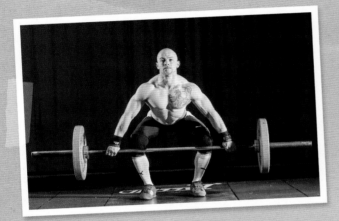
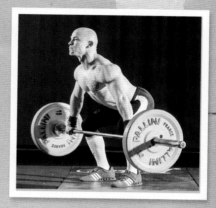

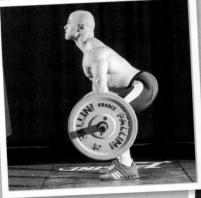
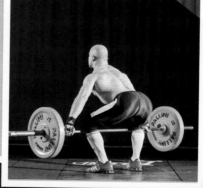

The knees flex just enough to allow the bar to pass.

The weight shifts toward the balls of the feet.

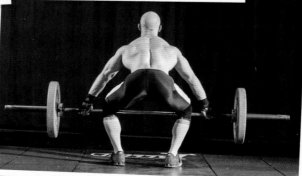

◉ Part 3—Transition

In this part, the movement slows down, so this part should be as brief as possible, even though it may last longer than it does in a clean. The transition is preparing you for part 4. The back straightens slightly to allow the knees to reengage under the bar, and the bar slides three-quarters of the way up the thigh. The weight shifts from the toes to the heels and finally to the soles of the feet. As for the feet, they should remain firmly in contact with the floor.

The slowing-down phase should be as short as possible.

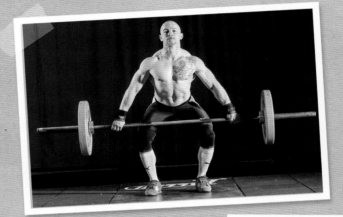

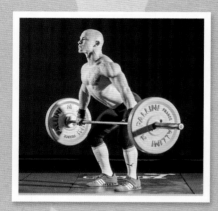

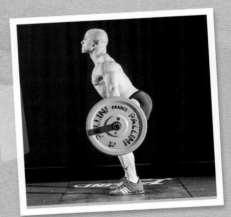

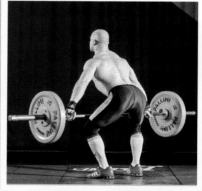

The knees reengage under the bar to prepare for the next movement.

The feet remain firmly in contact with the floor.

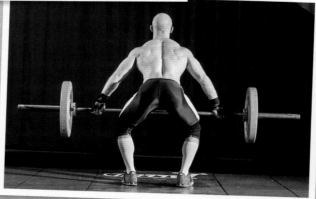

Part 4—The second pull

Just like the first pull, this part is driven by a large push from the legs that causes a simultaneous triple hip, knee, and ankle extension until they are all vertically aligned at the end of the movement. This movement drives the bar upward and helps the arms pull (lifting the shoulders and then the elbows) before they go under the bar. At this moment, the vertical height of the bar is of primary importance (it should be held as close to the body as possible). A large number of muscles are used in this part; practically the entire body is working to support the large-muscle groups.

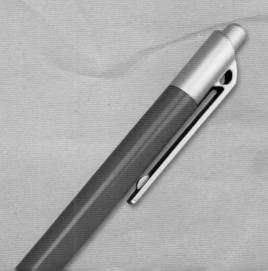

The second pull—part 1 of 3

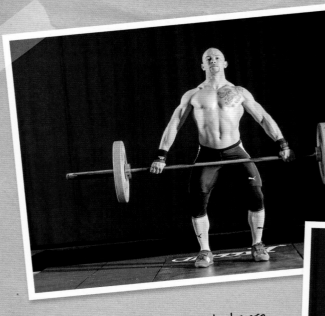

After the bar is past the knees, you are ready to accelerate it again!

Even at this stage, the lower limbs are still working to drive the movement upward through the hip extension.

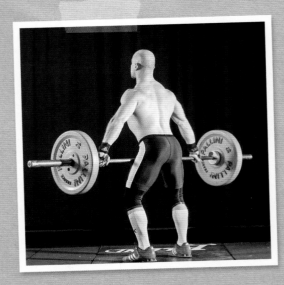

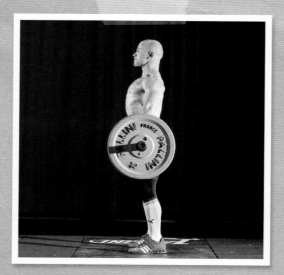

The second pull—part 2 of 3

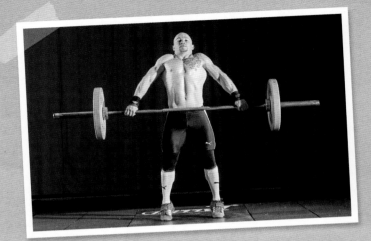

The shoulder shrug prepares the way for the arms.

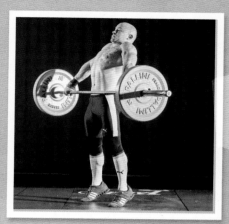

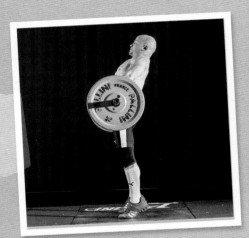

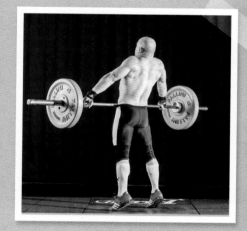

The shoulder shrug accentuates the height of the bar.

At this moment, the hips, knees, and ankles are in perfect extension.

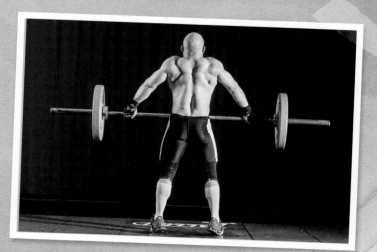

The second pull—part 3 of 3

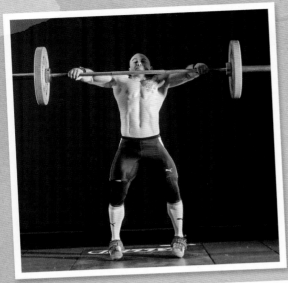

This triple extension does not mean hyperextension in the back; do not exaggerate the lumbar curve!

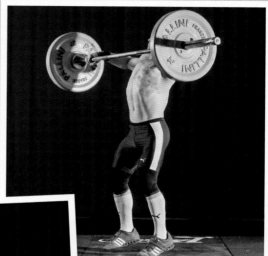

The elbows flex at the end of the second pull.

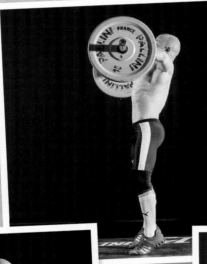

Depending on the weight, you may be able to lift your elbows more or less before sliding under the bar.

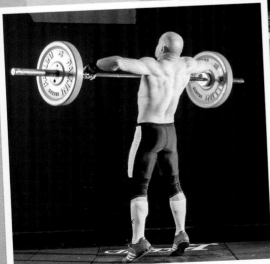

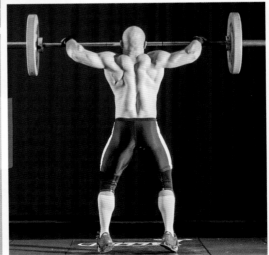

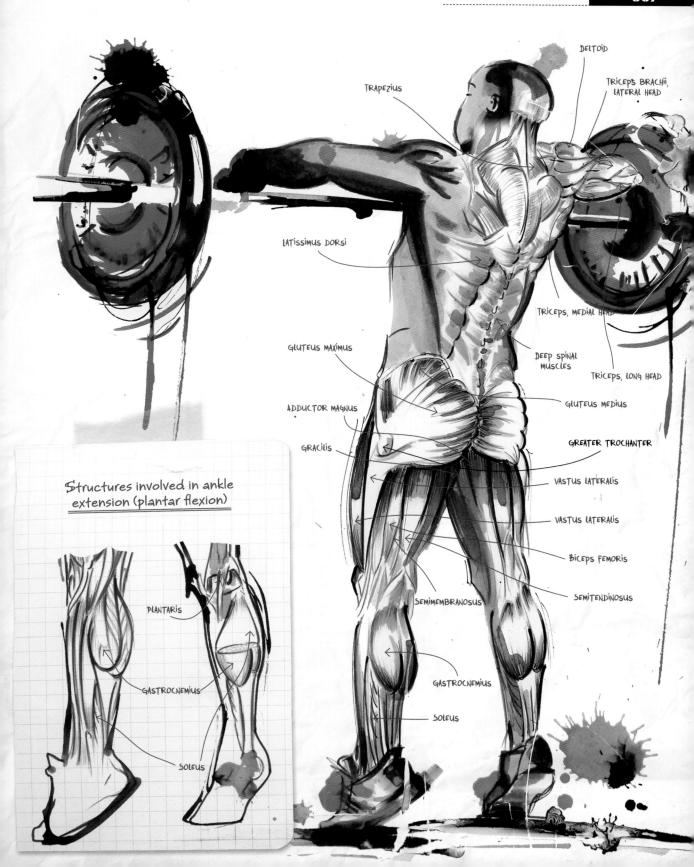

DELTOID

TRAPEZIUS

TRICEPS BRACHII,
LATERAL HEAD

LATISSIMUS DORSI

TRICEPS, MEDIAL HEAD

DEEP SPINAL
MUSCLES

TRICEPS, LONG HEAD

GLUTEUS MAXIMUS

GLUTEUS MEDIUS

ADDUCTOR MAGNUS

GRACILIS

GREATER TROCHANTER

VASTUS LATERALIS

VASTUS LATERALIS

BICEPS FEMORIS

SEMITENDINOSUS

SEMIMEMBRANOSUS

GASTROCNEMIUS

SOLEUS

Structures involved in ankle extension (plantar flexion)

PLANTARIS

GASTROCNEMIUS

SOLEUS

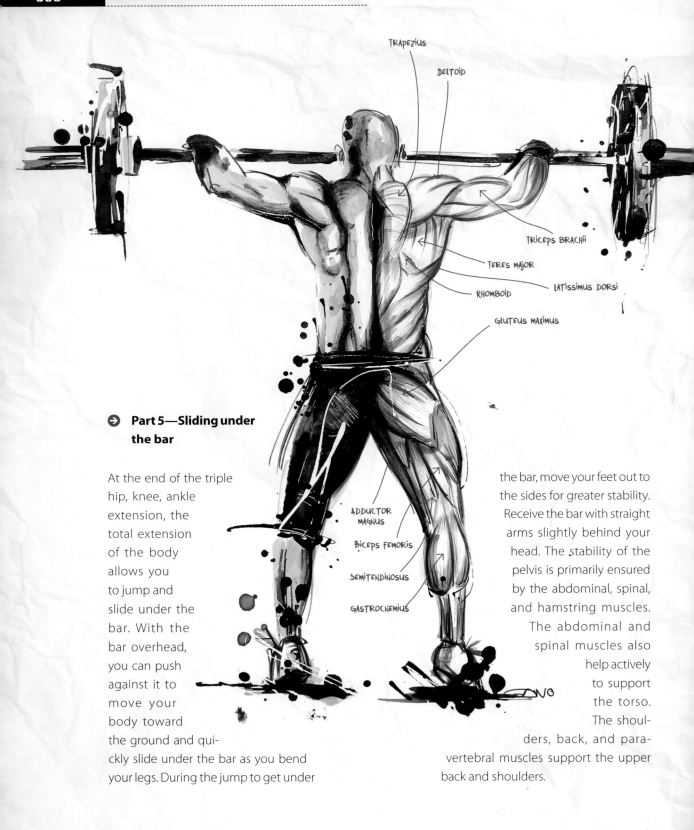

TRAPEZIUS

DELTOID

TRICEPS BRACHII

TERES MAJOR

LATISSIMUS DORSI

RHOMBOID

GLUTEUS MAXIMUS

ADDUCTOR MAGNUS

BICEPS FEMORIS

SEMITENDINOSUS

GASTROCNEMIUS

➲ Part 5—Sliding under the bar

At the end of the triple hip, knee, ankle extension, the total extension of the body allows you to jump and slide under the bar. With the bar overhead, you can push against it to move your body toward the ground and quickly slide under the bar as you bend your legs. During the jump to get under the bar, move your feet out to the sides for greater stability. Receive the bar with straight arms slightly behind your head. The stability of the pelvis is primarily ensured by the abdominal, spinal, and hamstring muscles. The abdominal and spinal muscles also help actively to support the torso. The shoulders, back, and paravertebral muscles support the upper back and shoulders.

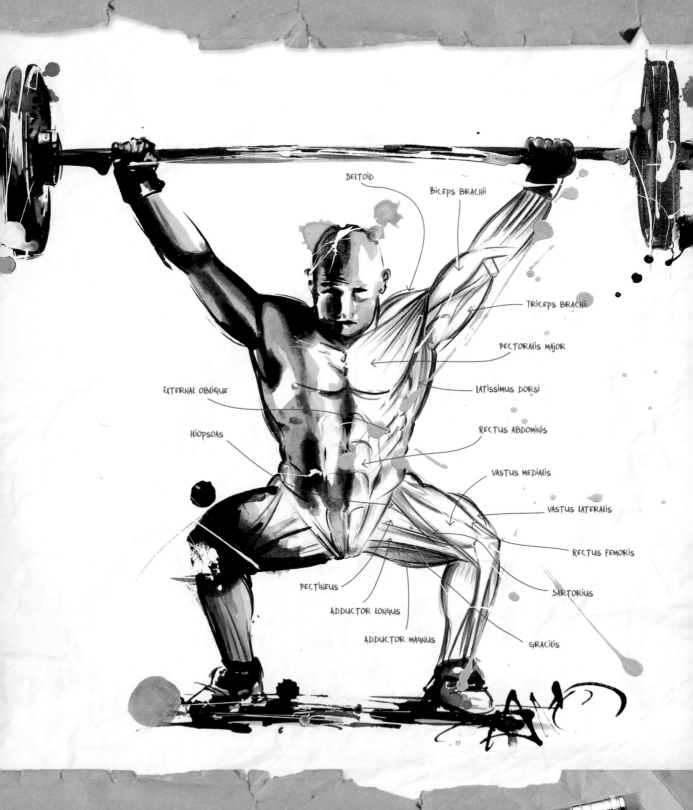

DELTOID

BICEPS BRACHII

TRICEPS BRACHII

PECTORALIS MAJOR

EXTERNAL OBLIQUE

LATISSIMUS DORSI

RECTUS ABDOMINIS

ILIOPSOAS

VASTUS MEDIALIS

VASTUS LATERALIS

RECTUS FEMORIS

PECTINEUS

SARTORIUS

ADDUCTOR LONGUS

ADDUCTOR MAGNUS

GRACILIS

➔ Part 6—Standing up and stabilizing the body

In the final part of the exercise, you must stand up with straight legs and bring your feet back to their original position while keeping your arms straight and the bar just behind the head. Of course, your back stays straight, and your gaze is high and fixed on a point just above the horizon. Do not relax control of your torso or your upper back and shoulders. Only after you are completely upright and balanced can you release the weight.

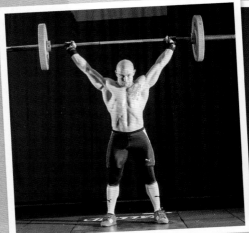

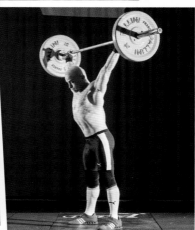

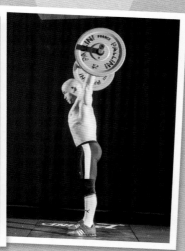

Keep your shoulders and torso firmly supported.

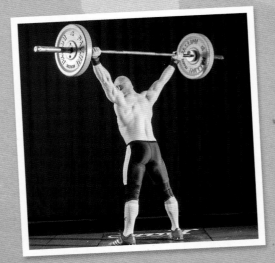

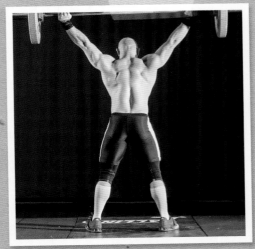

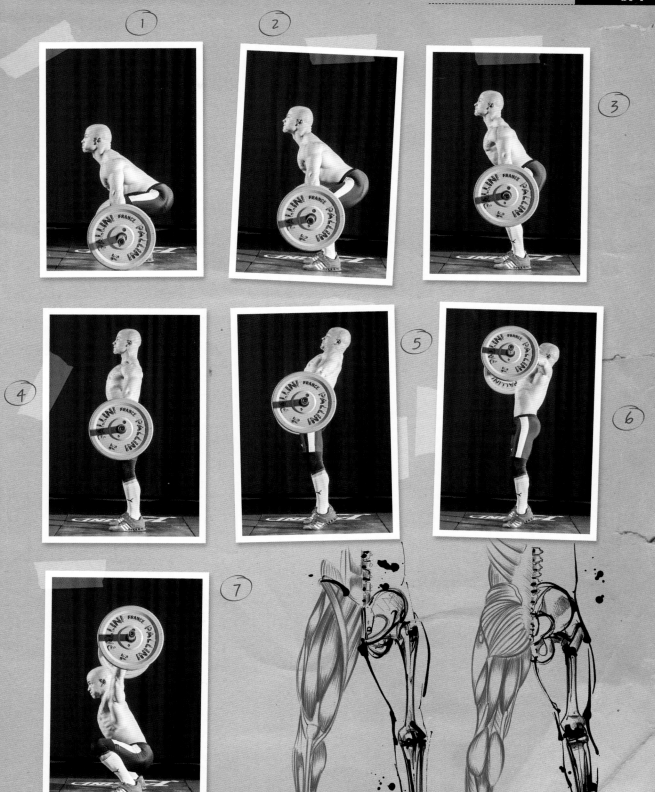

The shoulder complex

To understand the shoulder well, you have to consider its complexity: It is fragile, mobile, and adaptable, and it can easily be placed in dangerous positions. Worse, problems or inflammation in the shoulder joint can spread to nearby areas, through the ribs and vertebrae.

So taking care of your shoulders every day should be a priority. Do not perform hundreds of reps if you are not certain they are important or if you are not positive you are using correct form.

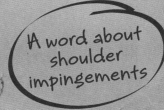

A word about shoulder impingements

The rotator cuff: a sensitive area

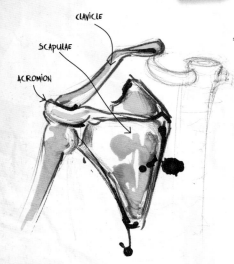

CLAVICLE

SCAPULAE

ACROMION

The rotator cuff suffers abuse in many situations. Injuries may occur after an accident, but they often result from repetitive movements that put the shoulder chronically in a bad position, causing generalized inflammation. When the glenoid cavity is not in harmony and is subjected to inappropriate movement of the shoulder, the head of the humerus can move, creating an impingement.

The more intense these impingements are or the more often they are repeated, the more inflammation they will cause in the rotator cuff muscles.

In fact, the tendons of the rotator cuff muscles pass between the glenoid cavity and the head of the humerus, so they can get pinched between the bone and the glenoid surface.

The glenoid cavity is composed of the acromion, the acromioclavicular joint, the coracoid process, and the coracoacromial ligament. The rotator cuff has five muscles: the supraspinatus, the infraspinatus, the teres minor, the subscapularis, and the long head of the biceps.

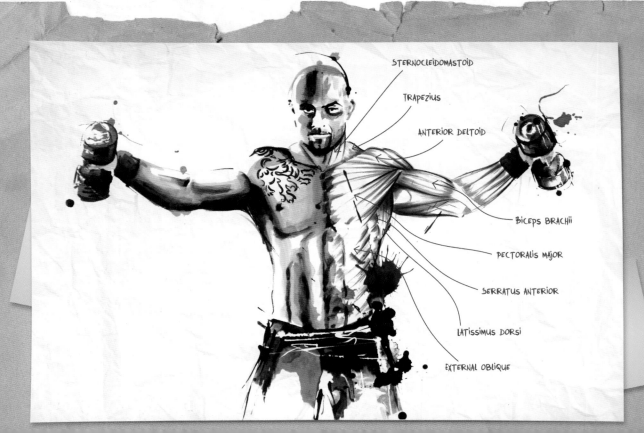

STERNOCLEIDOMASTOID

TRAPEZIUS

ANTERIOR DELTOID

BICEPS BRACHII

PECTORALIS MAJOR

SERRATUS ANTERIOR

LATISSIMUS DORSI

EXTERNAL OBLIQUE

The fragile, small shoulder ligaments

We have talked about the fragile muscles that power and protect the shoulder. But just under those muscles are many hidden ligaments that can be easily damaged by poor form! Never compromise your technique.

In practice, shoulder impingements happen at the end of a movement and are painful enough to interfere with proper execution of the exercise. They are the result of intense and repeated use of the joint, creating, because of faulty biomechanics, a rubbing and shearing motion between the bone and one or more tendons or bursa sacs. Exercises that are regularly performed incorrectly expose an athlete to shoulder impingements and are therefore potentially traumatic. Without going into too much detail, we will highlight the major ones.

Lateral raise

First, the dynamic lateral raise of a dumbbell (or a band) is generally done to strengthen the medial deltoid (see the photo of the exercise performed incorrectly). Many beginners make this technical mistake, which, if not corrected, will inevitably lead to injury. Proper form will have the elbow at shoulder height at the end of the movement. As much as possible, the elbow should guide the angle and elevation of the arm and not the wrist. This promotes the internal rotation of the arm and activates the trapezius muscle.

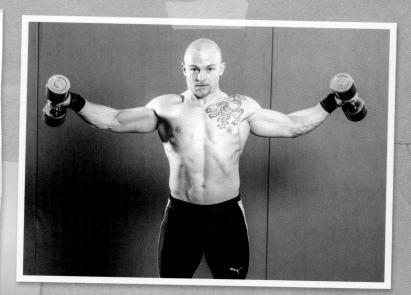

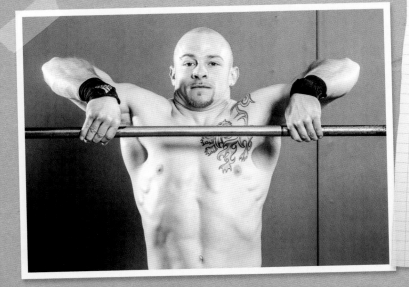

High pull

Another example that exposes the shoulder to subacromial impingement is the high pull, often used in upright rowing or in technical or semitechnical shoulder exercises.

More often, you can see this technical mistake made by athletes during a high intensity training workout, whether during cleans or rowing exercises with a bar or a kettlebell.

This error is unacceptable, and it should be corrected immediately.

A word about shoulder impingements

The humerus slides forward

Bench press

Finally, working the pectoralis major, especially in the most famous gym exercise, the bench press, whether with dumbbells or a conventional bar, if done with improper form can be dangerous for the stability of the head of the humerus. Often, devotees of the bench press prefer to use a wide bench for greater stability and a wide hand grip.

Lowering the weight to the chest drives the shoulder blades into the bench. Simultaneously, the shortening of the pectoral muscles forces the head of the humerus forward against the glenoid cavity just at the moment that the humerus needs greater mobility within the glenoid cavity.

This forward slippage can cause internal front shoulder pain.

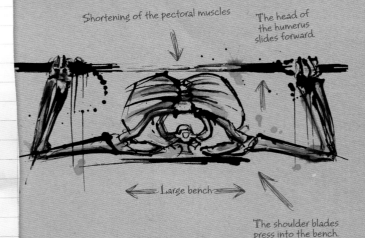

Shortening of the pectoral muscles

The head of the humerus slides forward.

← Large bench →

The shoulder blades press into the bench.

An anatomically correct bench press

In this case as well, mastering the basic technique for the bench press and using a few preventative measures will reduce risk of injury.

Using a narrower bench and a narrower hand grip and not lifting the heaviest weights possible are easy-to-follow strategies to make this exercise more comfortable anatomically.

If you are working with dumbbells, simply shorten your range of movement, which limits the shortening of the pectoral muscles and their primary effect on forward slippage.

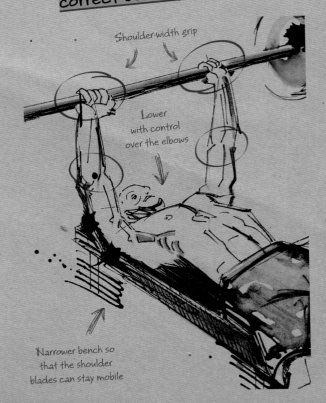

Shoulder-width grip

Lower with control over the elbows

Narrower bench so that the shoulder blades can stay mobile

WORKOUT - SNATCHES

WORKOUT 1 - SNATCH THE BURPEES

10 SETS, STARTING EVERY MINUTE:

3 SNATCHES FROM THREE-QUARTERS UP THE THIGH

6 BURPEES (PAGE 165)

4 MINUTES OF REST

3 X 1 MINUTE OF RUNNING, COVERING THE MAXIMUM POSSIBLE DISTANCE

RECOVERY: 2 MINUTES, AS ACTIVE AS POSSIBLE

WORKOUT 2 - LONG POWER

1 SNATCH AND 1 OVERHEAD SQUAT (PAGE 100)
EVERY MINUTE FOR 15 MINUTES

THEN 10, 8, 6, 4, 2 REPS OF EACH AS FAST AS POSSIBLE:
SQUATS (PAGE 89) AND BURPEES (PAGE 165)

WORKOUT 3 - PULL IN EVERY DIRECTION

3 X 5, THEN 3 X 3 SQUATS (PAGE 89)

AS MANY TIMES AS YOU CAN IN 12 MINUTES: 10 SNATCHES
FROM THE THIGH, 10 PULL-UPS (PAGE 143)

KETTLEBELL VARIATIONS

Weightlifting exercises can also be done with kettlebells. There are almost as many variations with kettlebells as there are for a regular bar. We will limit our discussion to techniques for snatches and cleans.

➔ Kettlebell snatch

You can do this exercise with a kettlebell in each hand, but a good reason to do this exercise instead of the barbell snatch is to only use one kettlebell to disassociate the left side from the right side. Start the exercise with the legs bent, the

back flat, and the chest out. Your other hand can hang freely, or you can rest it on your knee. Get ready for the triple hip, knee, and ankle extension while raising your torso and lifting the kettlebell with the first vertical lift.

The kettlebell should be as close to your body as possible throughout the exercise. Continue raising the kettlebell by lifting your elbow as you lift up onto the balls of your feet. Lift the kettlebell again to raise it over your head and straighten your arm as you flex your legs.

The kettlebell will be blocked by the thumb with the hand fully inserted in the handle.

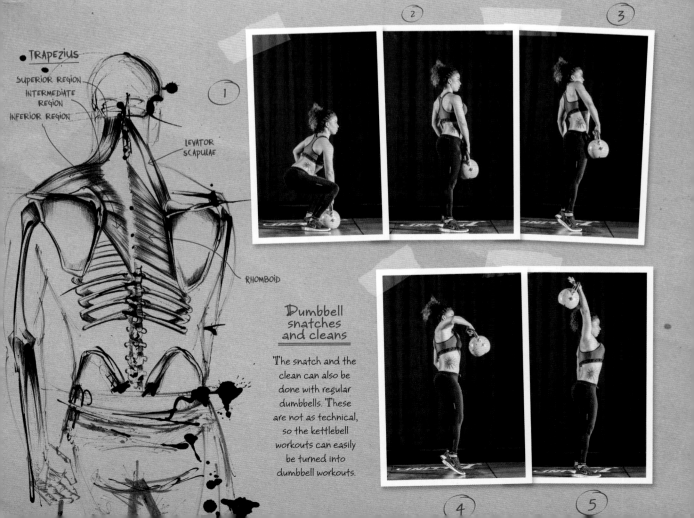

TRAPEZIUS
- SUPERIOR REGION
- INTERMEDIATE REGION
- INFERIOR REGION

LEVATOR SCAPULAE

RHOMBOID

Dumbbell snatches and cleans

The snatch and the clean can also be done with regular dumbbells. These are not as technical, so the kettlebell workouts can easily be turned into dumbbell workouts.

WORKOUT - KETTLEBELL SNATCHES

WORKOUT 1 - COLORADO SPRING

DO 5 ROUNDS AS FAST AS POSSIBLE:

400-METER RUNNING

20 BODYWEIGHT SQUATS (PAGE 89)

10 LIGHT KETTLEBELL SNATCHES PER ARM

WORKOUT 2 - LEGS AND SHOULDERS

DO 3 ROUNDS AS FAST AS POSSIBLE:

4 X 5 SQUATS (PAGE 89)

THEN

5 KETTLEBELL SNATCHES WITH THE RIGHT ARM

5 KETTLEBELL JERKS WITH BOTH ARMS IN A FRONT SPLIT POSITION

5 KETTLEBELL SNATCHES WITH THE LEFT ARM

5 KETTLEBELL JERKS WITH BOTH ARMS IN A FRONT SPLIT POSITION

20 TOES TO BAR (ON A PULL-UP BAR) (PAGE 185)

RUN FOR 200 METERS.

WORKOUT 3 - AMAZON FURY

EVERY MINUTE FOR 17 MINUTES:

4 ALTERNATING PUSH-UPS ON A KETTLEBELL

4 KETTLEBELL SNATCHES PER ARM

4 KETTLEBELL THRUSTERS WITH BOTH ARMS

⊙ Kettlebell clean

Like a kettlebell snatch, this exercise can be done with one or two kettlebells. This time, because you cannot control the kettlebell by putting your hand into the handle, you have to rest the kettlebell (or kettlebells) on the shoulders with your arm (or arms) bent. You must be careful to slow the movement before the kettlebell touches the shoulder (to avoid an injury that will put an abrupt stop to your set) by tightly squeezing the handle to stop the rotation of the kettlebell.

You can start with the kettlebells on the floor or up on blocks. As with the clean with a bar, the movement begins with a strong push from the legs that drives the extension of the hips, knees, and ankles. Keep the back straight as the weight moves upward. A shoulder shrug and then an elbow flex will propel the kettle-

bell (or kettlebells) upward so that you can slide under the weight.

Here is where this exercise differs from a clean with a bar: You have to rotate the kettlebell (or kettlebells) as you are pulling upward so that your grip changes from an upper grip to a lower grip, allowing you to rest the kettlebell (or kettlebells) on the shoulders. After the kettlebells are stopped and you are stable in a quarter-squat position, you are ready to start again. Although the height of the weight is not as important here as it is for a snatch, you still absolutely cannot allow the kettlebell or kettlebells to swing away from the body.

Depending on the workout, the kettlebell clean can be followed by a kettlebell jerk. The technical details for that exercise are the same as for the classic weightlifting version of the exercise.

Key technical points:

- Ankle extension
- Shoulder shrug
- Proper kettlebell trajectory
- Back in alignment
- Lower the kettlebell onto the shoulder with control

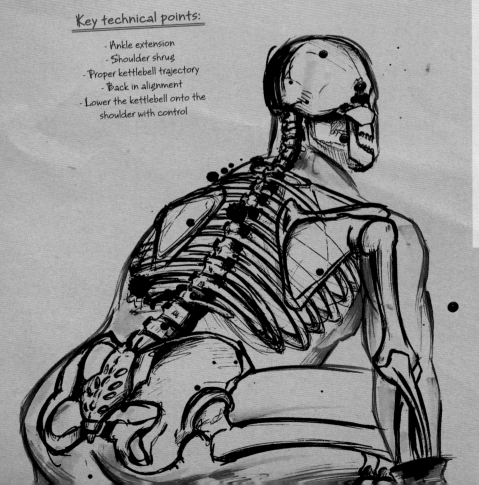

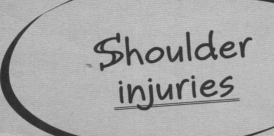

Shoulder injuries

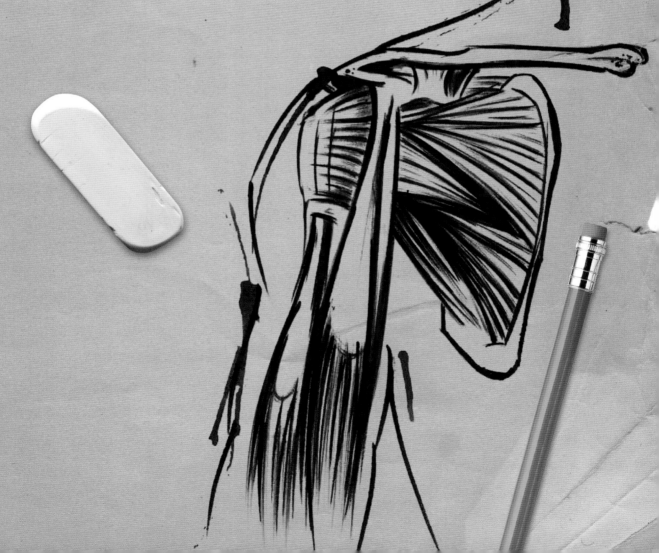

If not taken seriously,
inflammation in the shoulder
can eventually spread to all
the muscles in the shoulder.

①

Remember that the shoulder has great multidirectional mobility. This mobility comes at the expense of stability and strength. In fact, the humerus is locked into the glenoid cavity like a ball in a hole. It is held in place only by a complex and fragile system of muscles and tendons. As long as this system is strong and responsive, it protects the shoulder.

Most injuries happen during movements that recruit and exhaust the deltoids. These movements force the rotator cuff muscles and tendons to intervene with more strength than they have. The first risk is chronic inflammation, which can cause tendinitis to affect the muscles in the rotator cuff. But fatigue in the joint, if not taken seriously, can lead to serious sprains. The load on this mobile joint should be applied carefully. Very long sets of cleans can lead to overfatigue of the shoulder muscles and tendons, destroying all control in the joint and exposing the athlete to injury.

②

A typical example can happen during a clean: The supraspinatus tendon can be compressed between the head of the humerus and the roof of the joint created by the inferior surface of the acromion and the coracoacromial ligament. Inflammation generally begins in the bursa, which usually protects the supraspinatus from too much friction, and progresses to the supraspinatus, the infraspinatus, and the biceps brachii. Finally, the entire rotator cuff is inflamed, and just lifting the arm becomes extremely painful. Continuing to do repetitive movements despite pain may cause calcifications or tears that lead to irreversible shoulder damage.

No matter what, remember that pain is not acceptable:

- A limitation because of stiffness at the beginning of a workout should alert you to a problem. You can then do some stretching. If things do not improve, you should change your program.

③

- A limitation combined with pain you have not experienced before is cause to change your program immediately. You can choose from many exercises, so you can certainly find other ones that will not injure you. At the least, perform the exercise at a different angle while you wait for the inflammation to subside.

- An injury that happens while training should make you ask yourself what you have done incorrectly and what you need to change so that it does not happen again.

- Long sets are not well suited to complex exercises because fatigue interferes with motor patterns. Do complex exercises in short sets; exercises with simpler technique can be done in long sets. Keep in mind that some joints, such as the shoulder, should never be worked in long sets because of the potential for injury.

If you are
experiencing
pain or chronic
discomfort,
adjust your
training program.

The muscles of the rotator cuff, front view

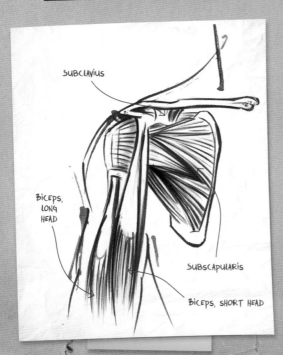

SUBCLAVIUS

BICEPS, LONG HEAD

SUBSCAPULARIS

BICEPS, SHORT HEAD

Hip joint

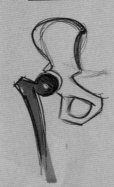

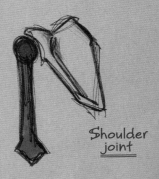

Shoulder joint

To understand the complexity and fragility of the shoulder joint, we can compare it to the solid hip joint. It is easy to see that the shoulder is as mobile as it is fragile; just because it can move to some angles does not mean that you should do it repetitively or with an exaggerated motion!

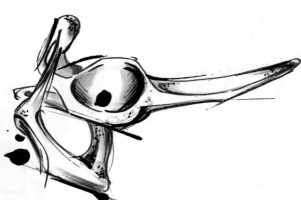

Side view of the scapulae showing the acromion, coracoid process, and glenoid cavity

The muscles of the rotator cuff, back view

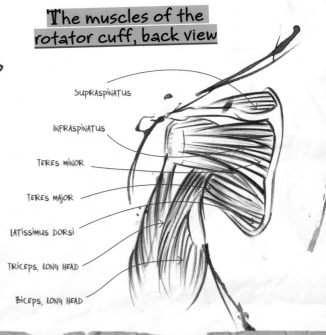

SUPRASPINATUS

INFRASPINATUS

TERES MINOR

TERES MAJOR

LATISSIMUS DORSI

TRICEPS, LONG HEAD

BICEPS, LONG HEAD

WORKOUT – KETTLEBELL CLEANS

WORKOUT 1 – CRAZY RUN

DO AS MANY ROUNDS AS POSSIBLE IN 25 MINUTES:

800-METER RUN

20 BURPEES (PAGE 165)

14 KETTLEBELL CLEANS

WORKOUT 2 – THE SEVEN MERCENARIES

7 ROUNDS WITH A MAXIMUM OF 3 MINUTES OF RECOVERY:

50 METERS OF FORWARD LUNGES (PAGE 140)

15 KNEE TUCK JUMPS

9 KETTLEBELL CLEANS

WORKOUT 3 – BROTHER JACK

EVERY MINUTE FOR 17 MINUTES:

TWO-HANDED KETTLEBELL CLEAN, 3 COMPLETE SQUATS (PAGE 89),
3 THRUSTERS (PAGE 103), 3 KNEE TUCK JUMPS WITHOUT THE KETTLEBELL

BENT-OVER ROW

This exercise can be done with a bar, with one or two dumbbells, or one or two kettlebells. This weightlifting exercise strengthens the posterior chain.

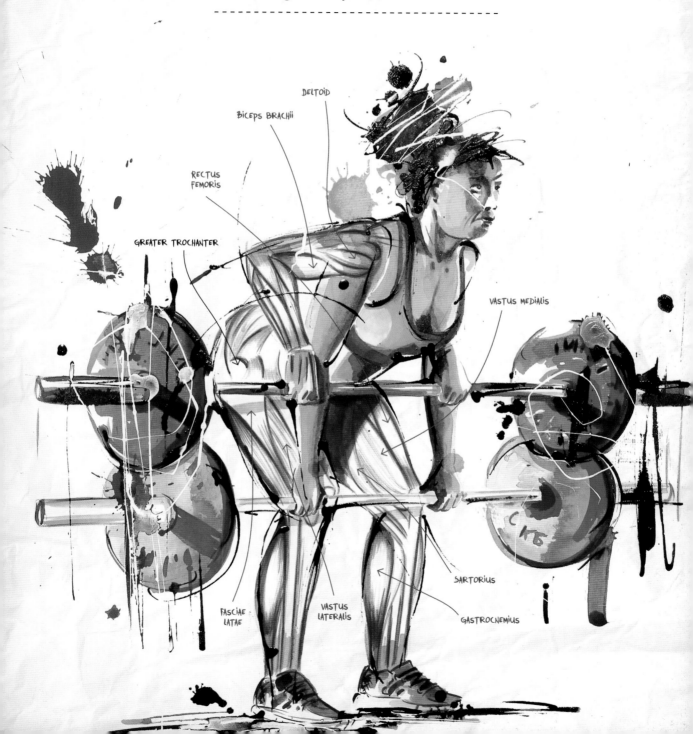

DELTOID

BICEPS BRACHII

RECTUS FEMORIS

GREATER TROCHANTER

VASTUS MEDIALIS

FASCIAE LATAE

VASTUS LATERALIS

SARTORIUS

GASTROCNEMIUS

Many muscles are involved in pulling exercises, including the latissimus dorsi, the erector spinae, the teres major, the teres minor, the infraspinatus, the rhomboids, and the trapezius muscles.

The pulling muscles are supported by the grasping and flexing muscles of the arms as well as parts of the shoulders.

An athlete's back may already be well developed because of the number of pulling exercises in a high intensity training workout. Because these exercises focus on whole-body movements and conventional methods, if they are not performed with excellent technique, they may not activate the deep muscles. For beginners, these elements enhance performance and are even more important to consider.

Think about this during active core exercises (see page 182) and in adjusting your posture.

So, before doing a pull, you must be sure your spine is held rigid in the extension. This position means that the kyphosis disappears, your chest sticks out, you pull the shoulder blades together, and you pull the shoulders backward.

This last activation of the rhomboids helps to maintain proper posture and causes maximal activation of the middle part of the trapezius.

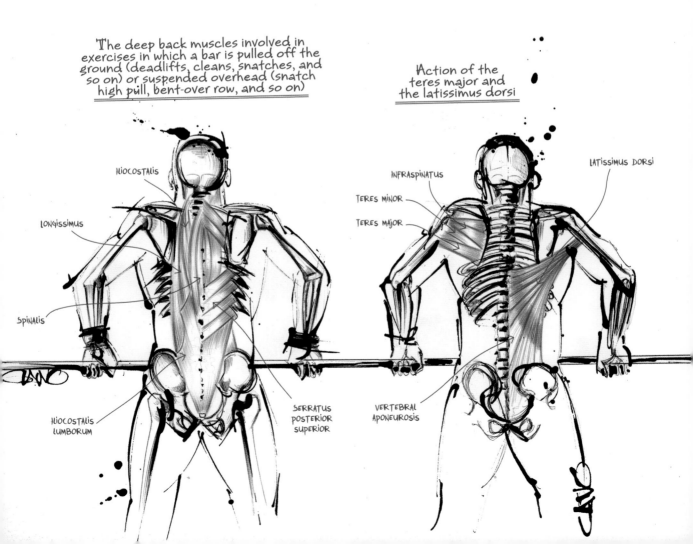

The deep back muscles involved in exercises in which a bar is pulled off the ground (deadlifts, cleans, snatches, and so on) or suspended overhead (snatch high pull, bent-over row, and so on)

ILIOCOSTALIS

LONGISSIMUS

SPINALIS

ILIOCOSTALIS LUMBORUM

SERRATUS POSTERIOR SUPERIOR

Action of the teres major and the latissimus dorsi

INFRASPINATUS

TERES MINOR

TERES MAJOR

LATISSIMUS DORSI

VERTEBRAL APONEUROSIS

The trapezius

Any pulling action involves a complex muscular chain that includes not only the muscles of different joints but also many layers of muscle. Do not forget those hidden muscles!

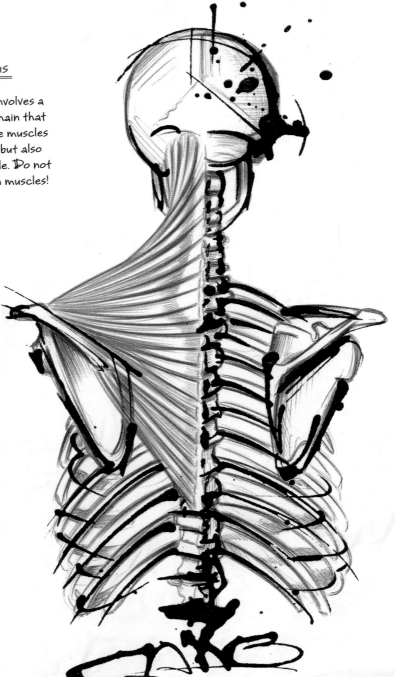

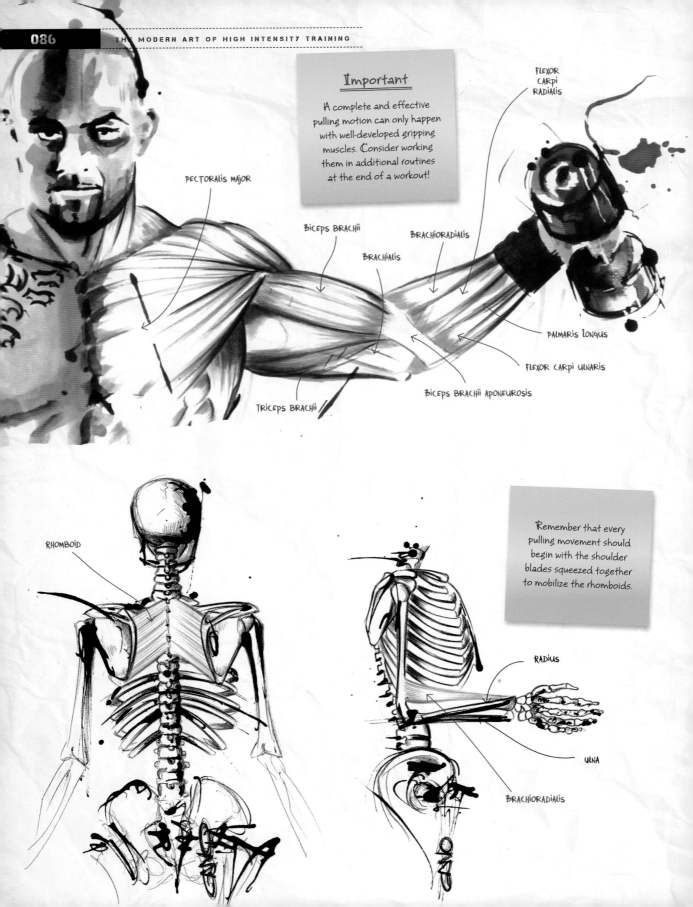

FLEXOR CARPI RADIALIS

Important

A complete and effective pulling motion can only happen with well-developed gripping muscles. Consider working them in additional routines at the end of a workout!

PECTORALIS MAJOR

BICEPS BRACHII

BRACHIALIS

BRACHIORADIALIS

PALMARIS LONGUS

FLEXOR CARPI ULNARIS

BICEPS BRACHII APONEUROSIS

TRICEPS BRACHII

Remember that every pulling movement should begin with the shoulder blades squeezed together to mobilize the rhomboids.

RHOMBOID

RADIUS

ULNA

BRACHIORADIALIS

This exercise may also be done with dumbbells or with kettlebells, in which case you should lean a little more forward and use a neutral hand grip (this can be adjusted throughout the exercise). You can also pull higher, with the hands reaching the side of your torso. The muscles recruited are slightly different from those recruited when using a bar.

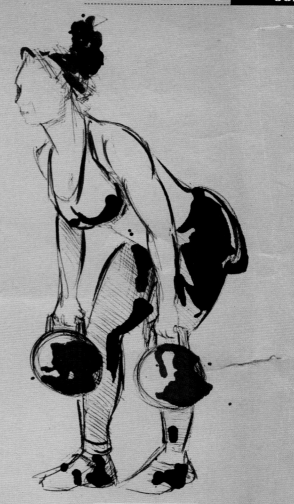

Technique tips

Lean forward with a slight bend in the knees to create a 90- to 145-degree angle with the torso and grab the bar with straight arms. Keep your head in a neutral position and in alignment with the spine. Get ready to pull by squeezing the shoulder blades together and sliding your shoulders backward. Bring the bar as high as your abdomen and then return to the starting position.

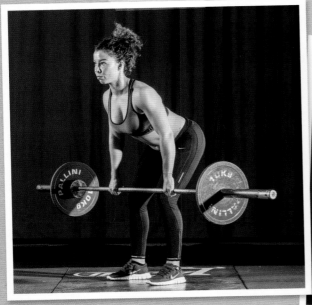

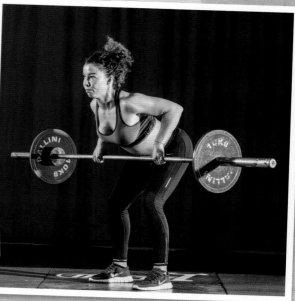

WORKOUT – BENT-OVER ROWS

WORKOUT 1 – MAGNUM

4 ROUNDS WITH 3 MINUTES OF ACTIVE RECOVERY BETWEEN ROUNDS:

400-METER RUN, 20 BURPEES WITH KNEE TUCK JUMPS (PAGE 165), 15 BENT-OVER ROWS

WORKOUT 2 – V-MAN

5 X 5 SQUATS (PAGE 89)

THEN DO AS MANY ROUNDS AS POSSIBLE IN 12 MINUTES:

8 JERKS (PAGE 47), 8 PUSH-UPS (PAGE 158), 8 BENT-OVER ROWS

WORKOUT 3 – FUNCTIONAL HYPERTROPHY

5 ROUNDS WITH 2 MINUTES OF RECOVERY:

5 BENT-OVER ROWS WITH HEAVY WEIGHTS, 10 SECONDS OF RECOVERY, 5 CLAPPING PULL-UPS (PAGE 148), 2 MINUTES OF RECOVERY, 6 CHIN-UPS (PAGE 143)

FINISH WITH 25 MAXIMUM WEIGHTED PULL-UPS (PAGE 143) IN LESS THAN 2 MINUTES

BASIC ATHLETIC EXERCISES

✳ SQUAT

The squat has figured in the debate dividing the Anglo-Saxon approach from the Mediterranean approach for more than 30 years. There are two schools of thought: On one side are conservatives from strength sports who believe that if you are not doing squats, you are not building the body. On the other side are the cautious athletes who are knowledgeable about alternative methods and prefer to limit the number of squats (especially complete squats) in their workouts. As always, the truth is a bit more complex, and each type of squat has qualities that should be considered.

- -

DIFFERENT TYPES OF SQUATS

As usual, the first point of disagreement concerns terminology. To simplify things, let us consider the half squat and the complete squat. In reality, a deeper discussion often reveals that the complete squat is compared with other squats. Worse, in the gym, we realize that most "experts" extolling the virtues of the half squat are in fact doing a quarter squat.

To summarize, people are comparing half squats and deep squats in theory, but in practice, these are quarter squats compared with complete squats.

The squat is a continuous movement that can be done to various degrees.

To be sure that we are speaking the same language, our approach classifies the different squats using a definition that leaves no room for interpretation.

- **Complete squats**: The athlete goes down as far as his or her joint mobility allows without going so far that the pelvis tilts backward. He or she goes low enough that the hamstrings cover the calves.
- **Deep squats**: The athlete goes down until her or his thighs are at least parallel to the floor (parallel squat) or even beyond.
- **Half squats**: any movement between 90 degrees of bend at the knee and a horizontal position of the thigh.
- **Partial squats**: any squat in which the bend in the knee is less than 90 degrees.

These four squats do not involve the same recruitment or adaptations, and by distinguishing between them, we can clarify the debate.

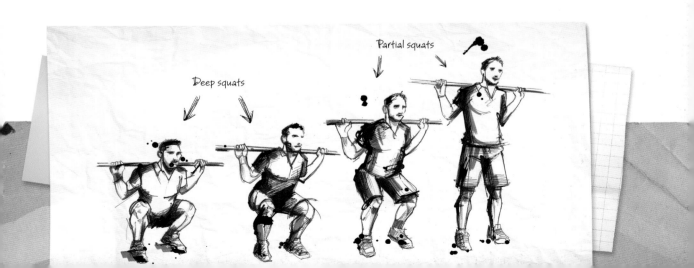

Deep squats   Partial squats

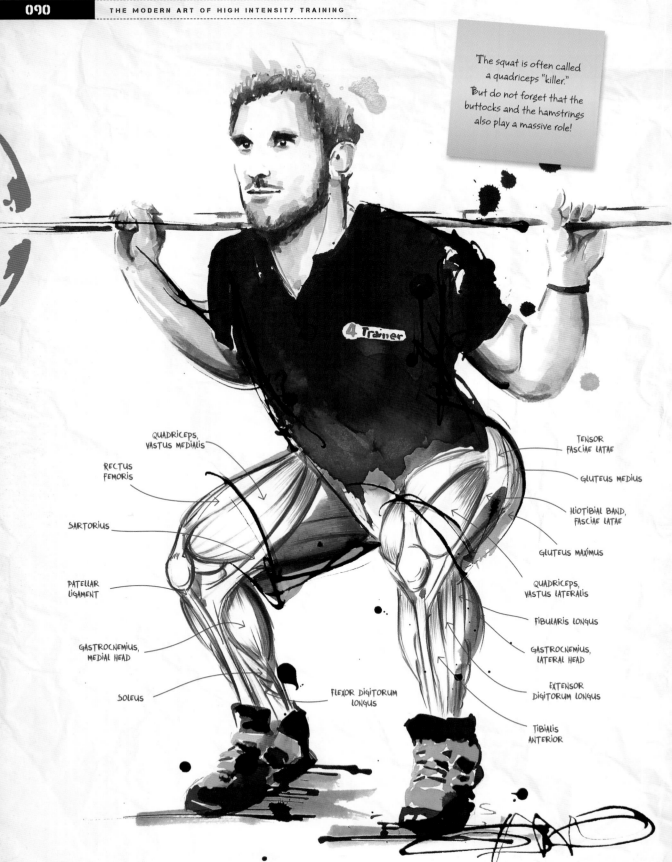

The squat is often called a quadriceps "killer." But do not forget that the buttocks and the hamstrings also play a massive role!

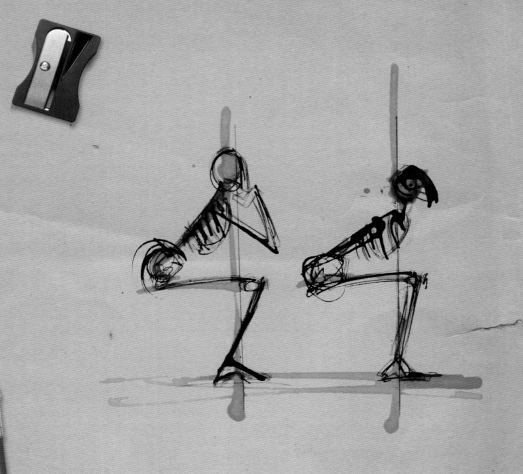

ANATOMY REMINDERS

In any form, the squat recruits more than 250 muscles: predominantly the quadriceps (vastus lateralis, rectus femoris, vastus intermedius, and vastus medialis), and the glutes (gluteus minimus, gluteus medius, gluteus maximus, fasciae latae, and its tensor), as well as the spinal muscles. Other muscles that help with stability are the hamstrings (semitendinosus, semimembranosus, and biceps femoris) and other leg muscles (triceps surae [gastrocnemius and soleus], tibialis anterior, extensor digitorum, and the fibularis longus and brevis). Finally, let us not forget the important role of core support and balance provided by the lumbar and abdominal regions.

HOW FAR SHOULD YOU GO DOWN IN A SQUAT?

Whether you are concerned with safety or with performance when doing squats, the depth is always a subject of debate. More often, the real question is how deep rather than how much weight should be on the bar.

In this case, an anatomical observation should help. The human body is conceived (and even optimized) to crouch down. Entire civilizations use a deep squat as a resting position.

See the drawing below. →

Let us be clear on this point. For a healthy knee, ankle, or hip, there is no reason not to do a complete squat. In 2001 Salem and Powers confirmed that stress on the knee does not vary between a complete squat, a half squat, and a quarter squat.

The problem grows more complex when the outside vertical load (and even interior load in the case of gaining body weight) increases. In this case, two problems can occur and should be monitored:

The vertical pressure that the weight exerts on the spinal column and especially on the discs. The human body is designed to lower into a crouched position but not necessarily while carrying three times its body weight. Using a heavier weight is part of making progress in your training, but you can use other methods to intensify a workout without having to use an unreasonable amount of weight on the bar.

The position of the pelvis is at different angles depending on the person. It cannot help but tilt backward, causing the spine to round forward.

Popular preventive practice recommends that this tilting is unacceptable and should never happen. But as long as the natural lumbar curve is maintained and the knees are in line with the toes, a deep bend is not a problem. Therefore, banishing deep squats is not necessary. Instead, the actual flexibility limit (squat depth) varies depending on the person. The limit is reached when an athlete no longer has control over the hips and the trajectory of the knees.

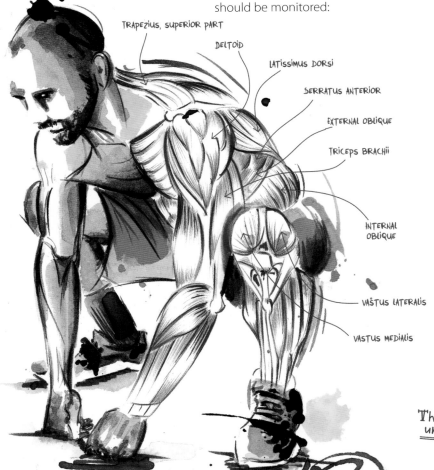

TRAPEZIUS, SUPERIOR PART

DELTOID

LATISSIMUS DORSI

SERRATUS ANTERIOR

EXTERNAL OBLIQUE

TRICEPS BRACHII

INTERNAL OBLIQUE

VASTUS LATERALIS

VASTUS MEDIALIS

The deep bend position is a universal resting position.

SQUAT MYTHOLOGY

At the margins of these semantic and anatomic considerations that clarify the debate lies the collective belief that a squat is more dangerous the deeper it is.

Several research teams put this belief to the test through experiments, and no serious study to date has shown the risk of injury to be greater in complete squats or performance gains to be lower than in half squats.

Despite this, many coaches and athletes consider partial squats less dangerous overall than deep squats. If you do not go very low, however, it is easier to load up the bar. Making progress in half squats is robbing Peter to pay Paul: You spare your knees the pressure, but you transfer that pressure to your spine, for a result that is not necessarily better. In fact, in 2012 Bryanton and colleagues found that progressing in squats has more to do with range of motion than with weight.

RANGE OF MOTION AND PERFORMANCE

The half squat is undeniably effective. As Zatsiorsky (1995) said throughout his career and in his book *Science and Practice of Strength Training*, few physical activities are done with a full range of motion.

Furthermore, gains in strength are optimized based on the range of motion that the athlete uses in training. So specific transfers should be expected during the first few degrees of flexion in the leg (even though more studies are showing gains over the entire range of motion) even when the work is limited to a partial range of motion (Massey et al. 2005).

Finally, according to Wilson in 1993, using very heavy weights increases progress in half squats by diminishing neural inhibition (though this argument ignores the risk to the spinal column incurred when using heavier weights).

It seems obvious that partial squats should have an important, but not exclusive, place in a training program.

As for deep squats, the study by Bryanton and colleagues in 2012 proved not only that they significantly increase muscle recruitment compared with partial squats but that the quadriceps are particularly sensitive to depth and that the glutes and hamstrings are activated even further when heavy weights are used.

The study also showed that the deeper the squat is and the heavier the weights are, the greater the effect is on an athlete's vertical jump. The posterior chain is activated during deep squats (with heavy weights, of course), and so it is no surprise that complete squats have a greater effect on jumping and explosive power in the lower limbs.

These two exercises appear to be similar, but they do not recruit exactly the same muscles.

The precise electromyographic analysis of various squat angles, as was done in 1994 by Signorile and colleagues, or even the measurements of muscular effort done by Bryanton and colleagues in 2012, provides us with precise information about the different structures recruited by different kinds of squats.

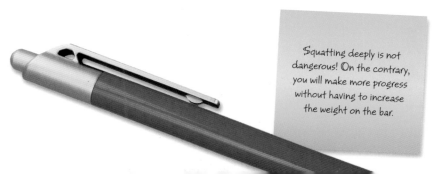

Squatting deeply is not dangerous! On the contrary, you will make more progress without having to increase the weight on the bar.

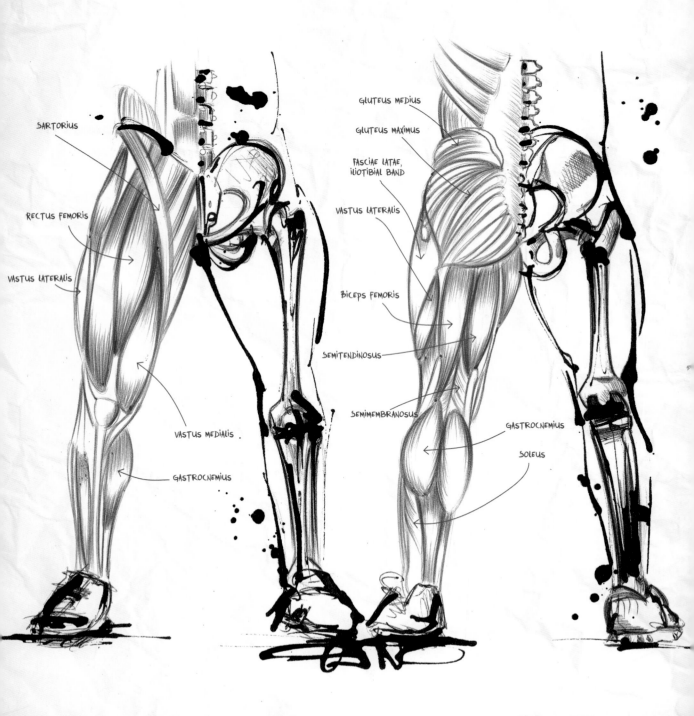

SARTORIUS

RECTUS FEMORIS

VASTUS LATERALIS

VASTUS MEDIALIS

GASTROCNEMIUS

GLUTEUS MEDIUS

GLUTEUS MAXIMUS

FASCIAE LATAE, ILIOTIBIAL BAND

VASTUS LATERALIS

BICEPS FEMORIS

SEMITENDINOSUS

SEMIMEMBRANOSUS

GASTROCNEMIUS

SOLEUS

SQUAT TECHNIQUE

The squat, whether complete or partial, is a technical exercise in which safety and effectiveness with perfect technique should come first. An athlete who lacks excellent technique may suffer from a lack of progress or even be injured. Ultimately, the entire training program could be affected.

- **The width of the hands on the bar**: Hands are placed on the bar just wider than shoulder-width, and the thumbs are locked around the bar.

- **The position of the bar on the back**: The bar should rest on the trapezius muscles and across the posterior deltoids, and the shoulder blades should be held together.

- **Stance**: The position of the feet may vary, but both sides should be identical. We advise you to use a symmetrical and comfortable stance.

- **Removing the bar from the rack**: Before starting the exercise, the bar should be on the rack, just below the level of your shoulders when standing. After the bar is positioned properly on the upper back, remove the bar from the rack by first slightly squatting down directly underneath it and

then standing straight up. After you are standing with a stable base, take a step back but stay close to the rack.

- **Head position**: The head should be in alignment with the spine, and the gaze should be fixed on an anchor point directly in front.

- **Flexion**: Put the knees and hips under tension at the same time to lower the center of gravity slightly. Keep your abdomen tight but do not exaggerate the lumbar curve. Lower the hips to the desired level for either complete or partial squats. The knees are in the same vertical plane as the thighs and feet. Keep your heels firmly on the floor.

- **Extension**: The extension of the knees, hips, and torso must be synchronized, and the knees should not be squeezed together. Come back up symmetrically in a smooth movement with no stops.

- **A critical point**: When the femur and the tibia form a 90-degree angle, muscle tension is at its highest level.

- **Speed**: You can use many techniques, but overall, the descent should be done with control. Any speed in this exercise should be done on the way up.

- **Breathing**: Take a breath just before the flexion and then exhale strongly at the end of the extension. Throughout the exercise, a coach should watch the position of the back and the control over the pelvic tilt. This supervision helps you maintain the natural curves of the spine (rounding the back is unacceptable, so if it happens, the spotter needs to take over).

Final reminders

Nevertheless, despite all the potential benefits of the squat in performance and prevention, those who speak out against squats are not completely wrong. In the guise of effectiveness, some coaches could be tempted to forego caution.

First, the age and experience level of the audience should be considered. Younger and inexperienced audiences should be educated about how to perform a squat properly. This caution does not mean that those people should never do squats, but squats are technical. More athletes are doing high intensity training without the needed technical experience; they must take the time to learn proper exercise technique.

Finally, the athlete should never use heavy weights for squats, whether complete or partial squats, until he or she has sufficient support and strength in the lower and upper body. The smartest way to begin is to build a solid foundation for the safe and effective practice of squatting for many years to come.

WORKOUT - SQUATS

WORKOUT 1 - FULL-BODY PUSH

5 X 3 CLEAN AND JERKS (PAGE 34), 2 MINUTES OF RECOVERY

AS MANY TIMES AS POSSIBLE IN 12 MINUTES:
5 SQUATS, 5 BENCH PRESSES (PAGE 120) AT YOUR MAX FOR 12 REPS

WORKOUT 2 - EXPLOSIVE SQUATS

5 X 3 SNATCHES (PAGE 60), 2 MINUTES OF RECOVERY

EVERY MINUTE FOR 10 MINUTES:
1 COMPLETE SQUAT AT YOUR MAX FOR 4 OR 5 REPS,
FOLLOWED BY A 60-METER SPRINT

WORKOUT 3 - FUNCTIONAL HYPERTROPHY

5 ROUNDS WITH 2 MINUTES OF RECOVERY:

5 SQUATS MAX, 10 SECONDS OF RECOVERY, 5 MAX VERTICAL JUMPS,
2 MINUTES OF REST, 6 PISTOL SQUATS (PAGE 111) PER LEG

END WITH AS MANY AIR SQUATS AS POSSIBLE IN 2 MINUTES.

FRONT SQUAT

A squat with the bar in front of the shoulders is the safest alternative to conventional squats.

It also happens to be one of the teaching strategies of basic weightlifting exercises. It can be easily combined with technical or semitechnical exercises such as different kinds of cleans or jerks.

This type of squat is also known to reduce intra-articular pressure in the knee by 15 percent without any loss of muscle activation compared with a conventional squat.

Doing front squats offers several benefits:

- Good activation of the quadriceps
- Easier alignment of the back
- Excellent neuromuscular activation, even when using a light weight
- Helps increase flexibility

This type of squat is still technical, and although we honestly recommend it, some people will not like it simply because they are not used to it or because they have some limiting stiffness in their ankles, shoulders,

or wrists. In this case, for immediate effectiveness and greater comfort while working out, choose a conventional squat.

If, however, you wish to improve your flexibility and coordination, take the time to introduce this type of squat into your workout.

Technique tips

The advice here is the same as that for doing a squat with the bar on your back. The only differences are the position of the bar and the way in which you hold it in place; you must lift your elbows as much as possible (ideally, your humerus should be nearly parallel to the floor).

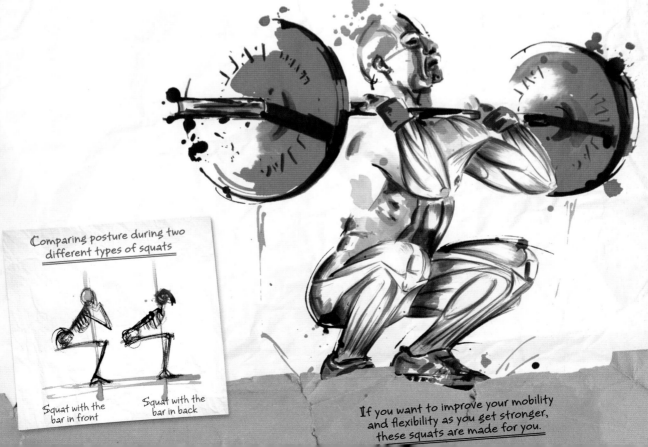

Comparing posture during two different types of squats

Squat with the bar in front

Squat with the bar in back

If you want to improve your mobility and flexibility as you get stronger, these squats are made for you.

Goblet squats

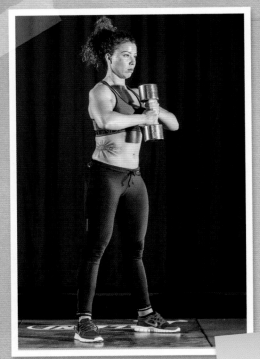

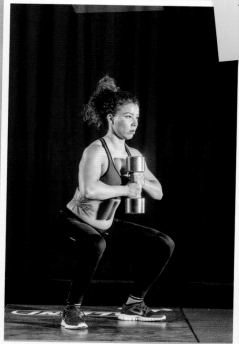

These squats can be done with a dumbbell or a kettlebell held against the chest, so they are called goblet squats.

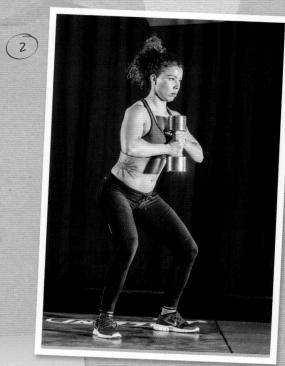

Goblet squats are particularly well suited for long sets.

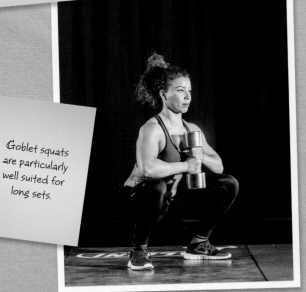

WORKOUT – FRONT SQUATS

WORKOUT 1 – MAXIMUM STRENGTH

3 X 5 FRONT SQUAT, 3 MINUTES OF RECOVERY MAXIMUM

10 X 1 FRONT SQUAT, 1 MINUTE OF RECOVERY MAXIMUM

WORKOUT 2 – FATAL COUNTDOWN

10 REPS THEN 9, THEN 8, 7, 6, 5, 4, 3, 2, AND 1 OF EACH EXERCISE:

FRONT SQUATS, BOX JUMPS, HANGING SIT-UPS

WORKOUT 3 – DOUBLE JUMP

4 X 3 CLEANS (PAGE 34)

AS MANY TIMES AS POSSIBLE IN 5 MINUTES:
6 FRONT SQUATS, 12 PULL-UPS (PAGE 143),
2 ROUNDS WITH 2 MINUTES OF RECOVERY

OVERHEAD SQUAT

This exceptionally postural squat is not only a foundational movement that reinforces the basic skills required for the snatch but also a powerful strengthening exercise.

Besides the usual muscle recruitment in a conventional squat, an overhead squat adds

- ➲ intense, dynamic core stability,
- ➲ shoulder control,
- ➲ strengthening of the stabilizing muscles around the spine, and
- ➲ stretching of the pectoral muscles.

Keep in mind that this exercise uses muscles that are much weaker than the large muscle groups used in a conventional squat. Therefore, you should moderate the intensity, both in the number of reps and the amount of weight used.

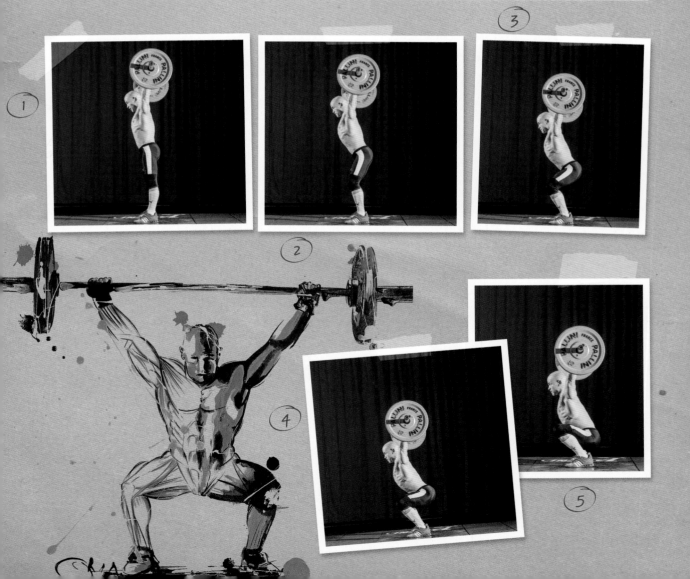

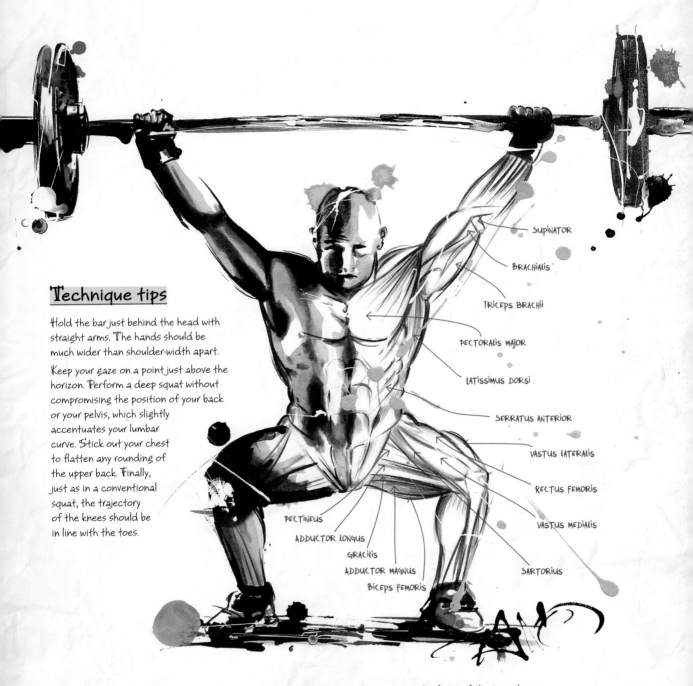

Technique tips

Hold the bar just behind the head with straight arms. The hands should be much wider than shoulder-width apart.

Keep your gaze on a point just above the horizon. Perform a deep squat without compromising the position of your back or your pelvis, which slightly accentuates your lumbar curve. Stick out your chest to flatten any rounding of the upper back. Finally, just as in a conventional squat, the trajectory of the knees should be in line with the toes.

SUPINATOR

BRACHIALIS

TRICEPS BRACHII

PECTORALIS MAJOR

LATISSIMUS DORSI

SERRATUS ANTERIOR

VASTUS LATERALIS

RECTUS FEMORIS

VASTUS MEDIALIS

PECTINEUS

ADDUCTOR LONGUS

GRACILIS

ADDUCTOR MAGNUS

BICEPS FEMORIS

SARTORIUS

Contrary to what you may have heard, the knees can go past the front of the toes during an overhead squat. What is not acceptable is allowing the trajectory of the kneecap to fall outside the vertical corridor formed by the big toe and the little toe. In addition to focusing on the upper body and using a wider foot stance than you use for a conventional squat, you must be careful to control the trajectory of your knees as you flex and extend.

WORKOUT – OVERHEAD SQUATS

WORKOUT 1 – WEIGHT WORKOUT

5 X 2 SNATCHES (PAGE 60), 2 MINUTES OF RECOVERY

AS MANY TIMES AS POSSIBLE IN 12 MINUTES:
8 JERKS (PAGE 47), 8 OVERHEAD SQUATS, 200-METER RUN

WORKOUT 2 – 21, 15, 9

21, 15, 9 REPS OF DEADLIFTS (PAGE 125) AND OVERHEAD SQUATS

WORKOUT 3 – OVERHEAD SQUAT AND BURPEE EXCHANGE

3 X 10 THRUSTERS (PAGE 103) THEN 3 X 10 JERKS (PAGE 47)
DO AS FAST AS POSSIBLE:
10 OVERHEAD SQUATS, 1 BURPEE (PAGE 165)
9 OVERHEAD SQUATS, 2 BURPEES
8 OVERHEAD SQUATS, 3 BURPEES
7 OVERHEAD SQUATS, 4 BURPEES
6 OVERHEAD SQUATS, 5 BURPEES
5 OVERHEAD SQUATS, 6 BURPEES
4 OVERHEAD SQUATS, 7 BURPEES
3 OVERHEAD SQUATS, 8 BURPEES
2 OVERHEAD SQUATS, 9 BURPEES
1 OVERHEAD SQUAT, 10 BURPEES

THRUSTER

Thrusters with a bar, kettlebell, or even with a sandbag are a complete movement that can help work on strength or metabolic endurance. The movement combines a conventional bar squat with a shoulder press. We recommend that you start with the bar in a front squat position to reduce the stress on the shoulder joints (read more about shoulder injuries on page 79).

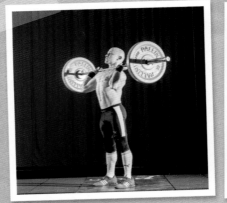

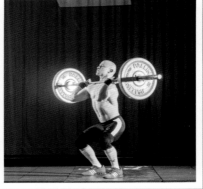

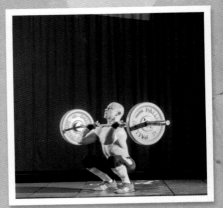

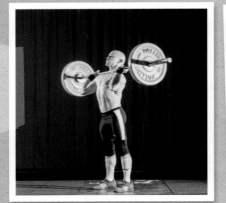

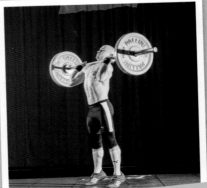

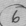

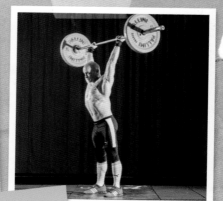

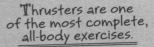
Thrusters are one of the most complete, all-body exercises.

Technique tips

This complete exercise combines the upper and lower body. Start in a front squat position, lower into a complete squat, and then come back up and go straight into a full shoulder press with your arms above your head.

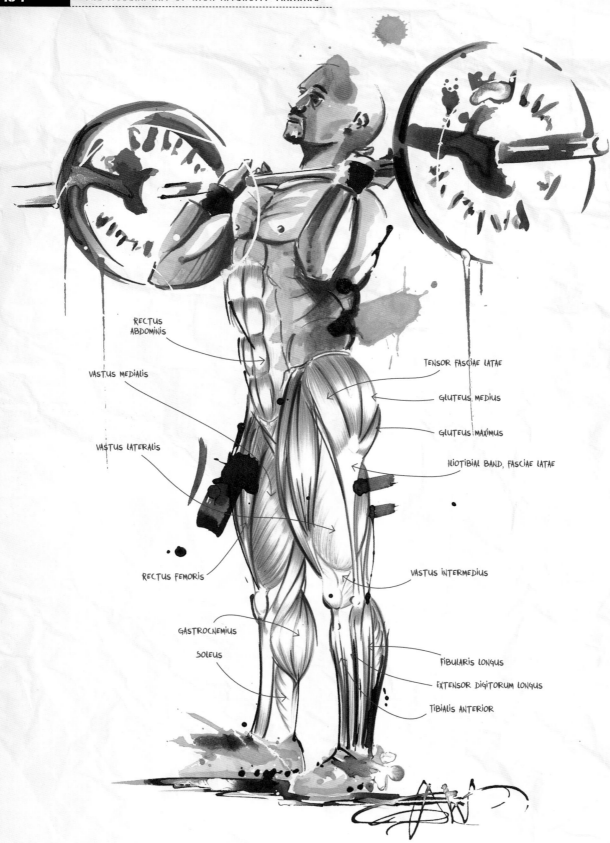

RECTUS ABDOMINIS

VASTUS MEDIALIS

VASTUS LATERALIS

RECTUS FEMORIS

GASTROCNEMIUS

SOLEUS

TENSOR FASCIAE LATAE

GLUTEUS MEDIUS

GLUTEUS MAXIMUS

ILIOTIBIAL BAND, FASCIAE LATAE

VASTUS INTERMEDIUS

FIBULARIS LONGUS

EXTENSOR DIGITORUM LONGUS

TIBIALIS ANTERIOR

Part 1: Bending the legs

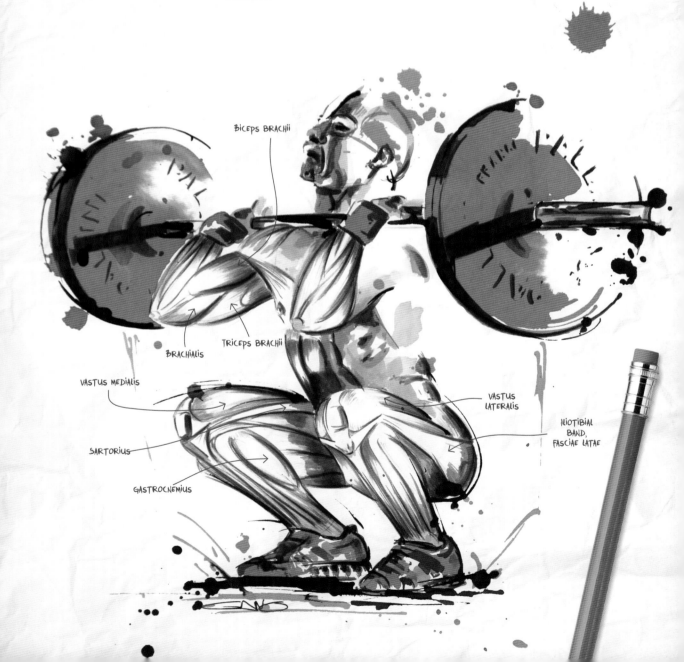

BICEPS BRACHII

BRACHIALIS

TRICEPS BRACHII

VASTUS MEDIALIS

VASTUS LATERALIS

ILIOTIBIAL BAND, FASCIAE LATAE

SARTORIUS

GASTROCNEMIUS

Do not allow the weight to control you! Stick out your chest and lift your elbows to avoid any rounding of your upper back. Even after long sets, be vigilant and hold your back straight to avoid potential injuries to the shoulders or spine.

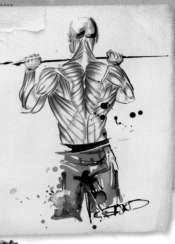

Stand up

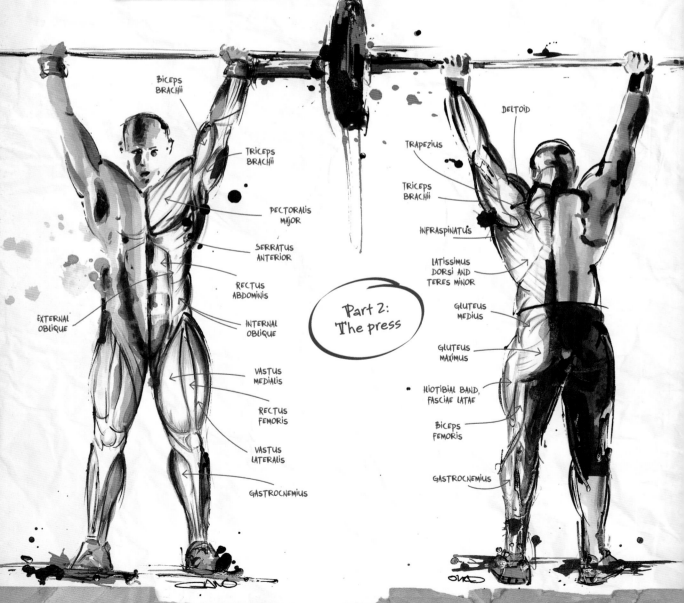

BICEPS BRACHII

TRICEPS BRACHII

PECTORALIS MAJOR

SERRATUS ANTERIOR

RECTUS ABDOMINIS

EXTERNAL OBLIQUE

INTERNAL OBLIQUE

VASTUS MEDIALIS

RECTUS FEMORIS

VASTUS LATERALIS

GASTROCNEMIUS

DELTOID

TRAPEZIUS

TRICEPS BRACHII

INFRASPINATUS

LATISSIMUS DORSI AND TERES MINOR

GLUTEUS MEDIUS

GLUTEUS MAXIMUS

HIOTIBIAL BAND, FASCIAE LATAE

BICEPS FEMORIS

GASTROCNEMIUS

Part 2: The press

WORKOUT - THRUSTERS

WORKOUT 1 - PUSH UP THE THRUST

40 SECONDS OF WORK AND
20 SECONDS OF RECOVERY:

ALTERNATE THRUSTERS AND
PUSH-UPS (PAGE 158).

YOU CAN CHANGE EACH SET BY USING A
BAR, KETTLEBELL, OR DUMBBELLS FOR
THE THRUSTERS AND BY ALTERING THE
HEIGHT OF THE FEET AND THE HAND
DISTANCE FOR THE PUSH-UPS.

REPEAT THE CIRCUIT FOR 20 MINUTES.

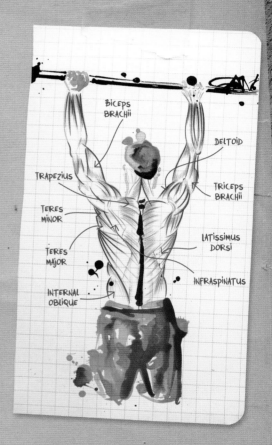

WORKOUT 2 - THE 15-15

5 ROUNDS:
15 THRUSTERS AND 15 BURPEES (PAGE 165)

WORKOUT 3 - THRUST THE BOX TO DEATH

21, 15, AND THEN 9 REPS OF BOX JUMPS, THRUSTERS,
AND THEN DEADLIFTS (PAGE 125)

ONE-LEGGED (BULGARIAN SPLIT) SQUAT

One-legged squats are particularly useful for athletes who are stronger on one side than the other and who need to rebalance their bodies. The exercise can be done with an exercise ball, a bar, or a kettlebell.

Technique tips

The technique used for the front leg to squat is the same as it is for a two-legged squat. You can also lift up the heel of your front foot at the end of the movement to isolate the calf muscles. The front foot should be placed on the floor far enough forward so that the front leg femur moves beyond perpendicular to the back leg femur and the front knee flexes to 90 degrees. The kneecap of the front knee will always go past the tip of the front foot.

Work on your balance

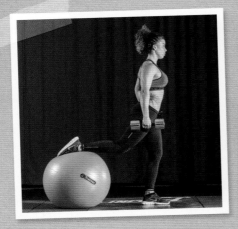
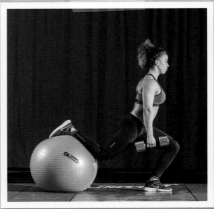
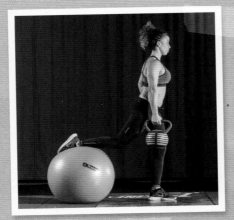
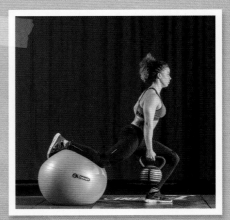
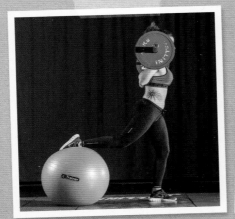
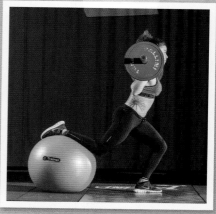

These one-legged exercises are not neglecting the nonworking leg; they just work that leg in a different way. Do not allow the back leg to rest. Instead, use this constant muscle recruitment to benefit and make more progress.

Lifting up onto the ball of your front foot during the upward movement phase of a one-legged squat is a great way to complement training your thigh with training your calf. This movement is more difficult, and you can do it isometrically (the heel stays lifted as the front knee flexes) or dynamically (the heel retouches the floor on each rep).

Achilles tendon

An Achilles tendon rupture can occur during training. Before workouts that involve a significant amount of running, take the time to warm up properly because an Achilles tendon rupture usually requires surgery and many months of recovery. Take care of the tendon and spend as much time stretching it as you do strengthening it.

Sensitive area

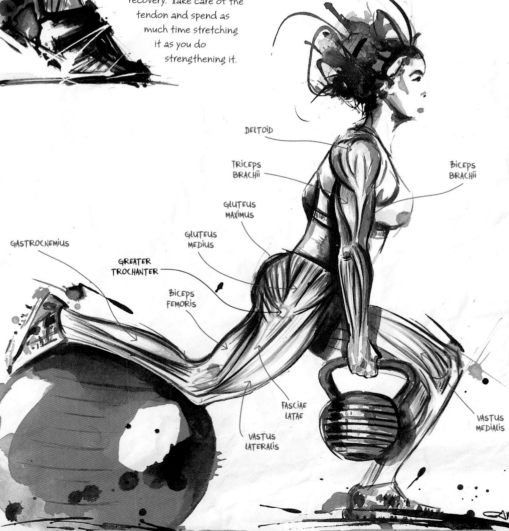

DELTOID

TRICEPS BRACHII

BICEPS BRACHII

GLUTEUS MAXIMUS

GLUTEUS MEDIUS

GASTROCNEMIUS

GREATER TROCHANTER

BICEPS FEMORIS

FASCIAE LATAE

VASTUS LATERALIS

VASTUS MEDIALIS

WORKOUT - ONE-LEGGED SQUATS

WORKOUT 1 - AZTEC

AS MANY TIMES AS POSSIBLE IN 20 MINUTES:

5 PULL-UPS (PAGE 145), 10 SQUATS WITH THE RIGHT LEG, 10 PUSH-UPS (PAGE 158), 10 SQUATS WITH THE LEFT LEG

AFTER 20 MINUTES, ADD A SET WITH THE LEFT LEG IF YOU DID NOT HAVE ENOUGH TIME TO FINISH A COMPLETE CYCLE (TO BALANCE THE RIGHT AND LEFT SIDES).

WORKOUT 2 - 10 ROUNDS PER LEG

20 ROUNDS AS FAST AS POSSIBLE:

5 PUSH-UPS (PAGE 158), 5 SQUATS WITH THE RIGHT LEG, 5 SIT-UPS, 5 SQUATS WITH THE LEFT LEG

AFTER 20 ROUNDS, ADD A SET WITH THE LEFT LEG IF YOU DID NOT HAVE ENOUGH TIME TO FINISH A COMPLETE CYCLE (TO BALANCE THE RIGHT AND LEFT SIDES).

WORKOUT 3 - E MAN

5 X 5 FRONT SQUATS (PAGE 97)

THEN AS MANY ROUNDS AS POSSIBLE IN 12 MINUTES:
8 JERKS (PAGE 47), 8 SQUATS WITH THE RIGHT LEG,
8 BENT-OVER ROWS (PAGE 83), 8 SQUATS WITH THE LEFT LEG

PISTOL SQUAT (AIR SQUAT ON ONE LEG)

These squats are often not performed because of the tension they place on the tendons. Indeed, we do not recommend them for heavy athletes or for beginners. The loss of control because of the difficulty of this exercise can cause inflammation, especially in the patellar tendon, and eventually lead to instability in the joint. More than ever, we advise you not to attempt this exercise unless you are strong enough and have sufficient experience to do it with perfect technique. You can reduce the load by using a strap or a band.

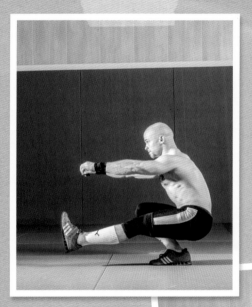
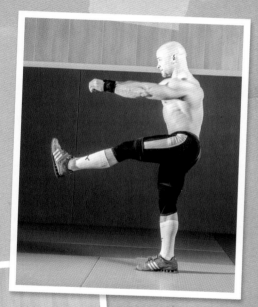
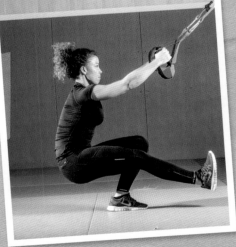

Pistol squats, if they are not done too often, are effective. Ideally, they should be used in bodyweight workouts, such as during vacation when you do not have access to gym equipment.

Technique tips

Right from the start, establish a counterweight by straightening your arms in front of your body. Stick out your chest to keep your posture as straight as possible throughout the exercise. Lift your head and fix your gaze on a point just above the horizon. Keep your eyes focused on that point throughout the exercise. Begin to lower your body on one leg while keeping the other leg in front of you and as straight as possible. To be successful, this exercise requires hamstring flexibility and strong hip flexors.

As you lower your body, keep the trajectory of the bending knee straight; it should not track outward (valgus) or inward (varus). Exhale as you rise up, pushing forcefully against the foot on the floor with your weight slightly toward the heel.

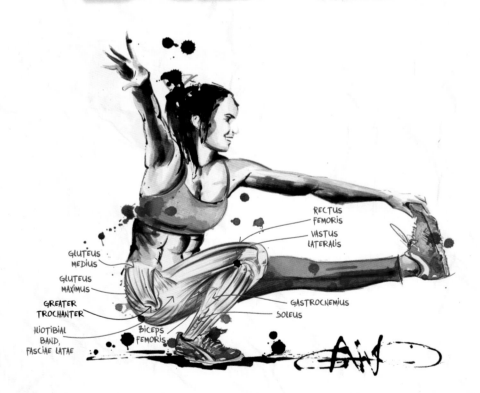

GLUTEUS
MEDIUS

GLUTEUS
MAXIMUS

GREATER
TROCHANTER

ILIOTIBIAL
BAND,
FASCIAE LATAE

BICEPS
FEMORIS

RECTUS
FEMORIS

VASTUS
LATERALIS

GASTROCNEMIUS

SOLEUS

Avoid
valgus
and varus
at all costs.

WORKOUT — PISTOL SQUATS

WORKOUT 1 — INCA

AS MANY TIMES AS POSSIBLE IN 20 MINUTES:

5 BURPEES (PUSH-UP AND KNEE TUCK, PAGE 165)

5 PISTOL SQUATS ON THE LEFT LEG

15 PULL-UPS (PAGE 143)

5 PISTOL SQUATS ON THE RIGHT LEG

AFTER 20 MINUTES, ADD A SET ON THE RIGHT LEG IF
YOU DID NOT HAVE ENOUGH TIME TO FINISH A COMPLETE
CYCLE (TO BALANCE THE RIGHT AND LEFT SIDES).

WORKOUT 2 — 36

5 X 3 CLEANS (PAGE 34), 2 SQUATS (PAGE 89), 1 JERK (PAGE 47)

THEN, AS MANY TIMES AS POSSIBLE IN 12 MINUTES:
12 PISTOL SQUATS, 12 PUSH-UPS (PAGE 158). ALTERNATE LEGS ON
EACH SET OF PISTOL SQUATS AND ADD A SET AT THE END OF THE
WORKOUT TO BALANCE THE LEFT AND RIGHT SIDES IF NECESSARY.

WORKOUT 3 — RUSSIAN ROULETTE

2 X 10 OVERHEAD SQUATS (PAGE 100)

3 X 3 SNATCHES (PAGE 60), 4 X 1 SNATCH

EVERY MINUTE ON THE MINUTE FOR 20 MINUTES:
3 PISTOL SQUATS, ONE-LEGGED BOX JUMP. CHANGE LEGS EVERY SET.

WORKOUT — MIXED SQUATS

WORKOUT 1 — SQUAT LIKE I

5 X 1 REP OVERHEAD SQUAT (PAGE 100), 30 SECONDS OF RECOVERY MAXIMUM

5 X 1 REP FRONT SQUAT (PAGE 97), 30 SECONDS OF RECOVERY MAXIMUM

5 X 1 REP SQUAT (PAGE 89), 30 SECONDS OF RECOVERY MAXIMUM

5 X 1 REP MAXIMUM VERTICAL JUMPS, 30 SECONDS OF RECOVERY MAXIMUM

ADDITION FOR THE END OF THE WORKOUT: 5 MINUTES OF ABDOMINAL EXERCISES WITH NO REST, CHANGE EXERCISES EVERY 15 SECONDS

WORKOUT 2 — PULL IT LIKE U SQUAT

3 X 10 FULL PULL-UPS (PAGE 143) USING A BAND ALTERNATED WITH 3 X 10 ONE-LEGGED SQUATS ALTERNATING LEGS (PAGE 108). RECOVERY BETWEEN SETS: 1 MINUTE

AS MANY TIMES AS POSSIBLE IN 5 MINUTES: 3 THRUSTERS (PAGE 103), 5 BURPEES (PAGE 165)

RECOVERY: LOW INTENSITY RUN FOR 3 MINUTES

AS MANY TIMES AS POSSIBLE IN 5 MINUTES: 3 FRONT SQUATS (PAGE 97), 5 KETTLEBELL SWINGS (PAGE 128)

RECOVERY: LOW INTENSITY RUN FOR 3 MINUTES

1,500-METER FAST RUN

WORKOUT 3 — GET SOME LEGS

5 FRONT SQUATS (AT YOUR 5-REP MAX) (PAGE 97), 10 SECONDS OF RECOVERY, 5 SQUATS (PAGE 89), 2 MINUTES OF RECOVERY, 6 ONE-LEGGED SQUATS ALTERNATING LEGS (PAGE 108), 2 MINUTES OF RECOVERY, 5 ROUNDS

15-MINUTE LOW INTENSITY RUN

WORKOUT 4 — CHARIOTS OF FIRE

3 FRONT SQUATS (PAGE 97) AT 60 PERCENT OF MAXIMUM, THEN 3 AT 70 PERCENT OF MAXIMUM

3 X 6 AT 75 PERCENT OF MAXIMUM, 1 MINUTE OF RECOVERY

THRUSTERS (PAGE 103) IN 1, 2, 3, 4, 5 REPS

AFTER EACH SET: 4 BURPEES (PAGE 165), 4 CLAPPING PULL-UPS (PAGE 148), 4 ONE-LEGGED SQUATS (PAGE 108)

LANDMINE SQUAT

This type of squat is valuable, because it allows you to focus the work on one side at a time, reduce the pressure of the bar on the shoulders, and limit the risks inherent to squats done in intense training.

Landmine squats can be done in many ways:

- With one or two bars (pushed together or one side at a time)

- With or without a shoulder press

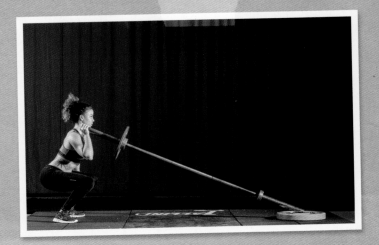

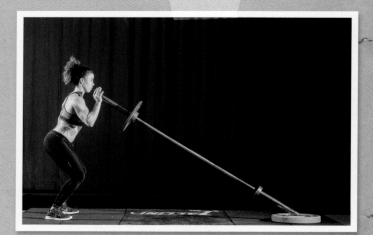

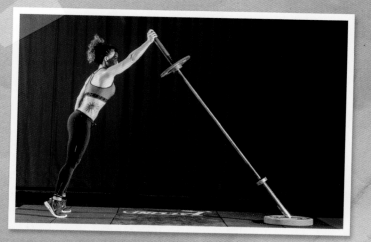

Technique tips

Grab the bar in one hand with the arm fully bent. Face the bar (no rotation is allowed) and perform a conventional squat. Landmine squats differ from normal squats in that you lean slightly forward. This position removes some load from your back, but it requires greater ankle flexibility to be able to reach a full squat position without the heels coming off the floor. As you come up, combine the hip extension with an arm extension (as in a thruster). Eventually, to complete the movement, you can add on by lifting up onto the balls of your feet before switching the bar to the other hand and starting the rep on the other side.

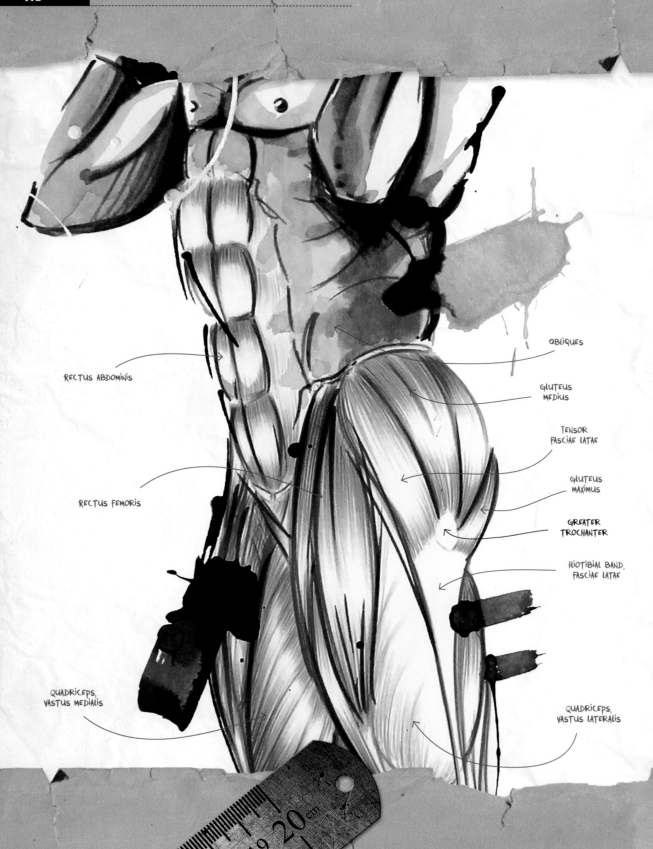

RECTUS ABDOMINIS

OBLIQUES

GLUTEUS MEDIUS

TENSOR FASCIAE LATAE

RECTUS FEMORIS

GLUTEUS MAXIMUS

GREATER TROCHANTER

ILIOTIBIAL BAND, FASCIAE LATAE

QUADRICEPS, VASTUS MEDIALIS

QUADRICEPS, VASTUS LATERALIS

LANDMINE OBLIQUES

This exercise is often combined with oblique work using torso rotations.

Many techniques are available, but we recommend the one that protects your back.

Technique tips

Grab the bar with both hands (one above the other; change hand grip on every rep) and then bring your hands to one of your hips. The back remains straight throughout the movement, and the chest is open with the head pulled up. As you pivot, keep your feet as parallel as possible to prevent the knee from pulling to the inside or outside. Follow these same instructions and bend your arms as you bring the bar to the other hip and reverse the position of the legs.

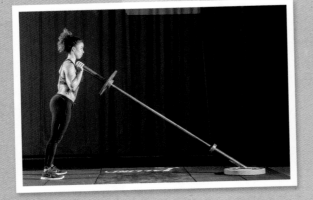

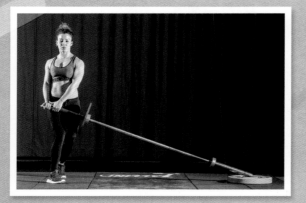

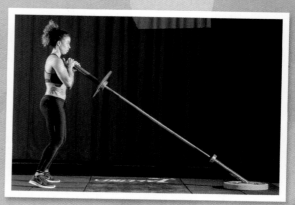

Although this is a complete exercise, you should focus on the abdominal muscles. Pull in the abdomen, control the forward tilt of the pelvis, squeeze the glutes, and tighten the pelvic floor.

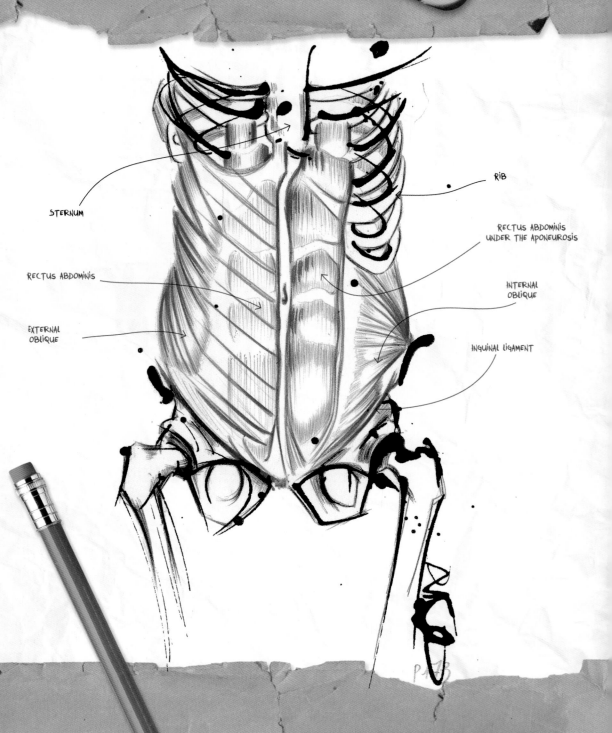

STERNUM

RIB

RECTUS ABDOMINIS UNDER THE APONEUROSIS

RECTUS ABDOMINIS

INTERNAL OBLIQUE

EXTERNAL OBLIQUE

INGUINAL LIGAMENT

WORKOUT – LANDMINE SQUATS

WORKOUT 1 – 180 DWARFS

20, 16, 12, 8, 4 REPS OF ALTERNATING HANDS LANDMINE SQUATS, ALTERNATING HANDS PRESSES, LANDMINE OBLIQUES

WORKOUT 2 – HEAVY DUTY

5 ROUNDS, AS MANY TIMES AS POSSIBLE IN 3 MINUTES:

10 LANDMINE OBLIQUES AT 50 PERCENT OF MAX SPEED, 10 JERKS (PAGE 47), 10 LANDMINE OBLIQUES AT 50 PERCENT OF MAX SPEED, 10 THRUSTERS (PAGE 103). RECOVERY: 2 MINUTES

WORKOUT 3 – 30 SECONDS OF HAPPINESS

10 ROUNDS: 4 CLEANS (PAGE 34), 30 SECONDS OF REST, 10 LANDMINE OBLIQUES WITH THE BAR AT MAX SPEED, 30 SECONDS OF REST, 10 LANDMINE SQUATS WITH TWO BARS, 30 SECONDS OF REST, 10 LANDMINE OBLIQUES WITH THE BAR AT MAX SPEED, 30 SECONDS OF REST

✖ BENCH PRESS

In this exercise, lie on a bench and grasp a bar with a shoulder-width grip. The exercise begins with the bar held over the chest with the elbows fully extended. Lower the bar and pause for a moment as the bar touches the chest and then push the bar back up until the elbows are straight. A bench press recruits the pectoralis major and minor, the triceps brachii, and the anterior deltoid. The stabilizing muscles around the shoulder blades (trapezius, rhomboid, levator scapulae, and serratus) as well as the rotator cuff (teres major, supraspinatus, infraspinatus, and subscapularis) primarily help with guidance and mastery of the movement (posture and core support).

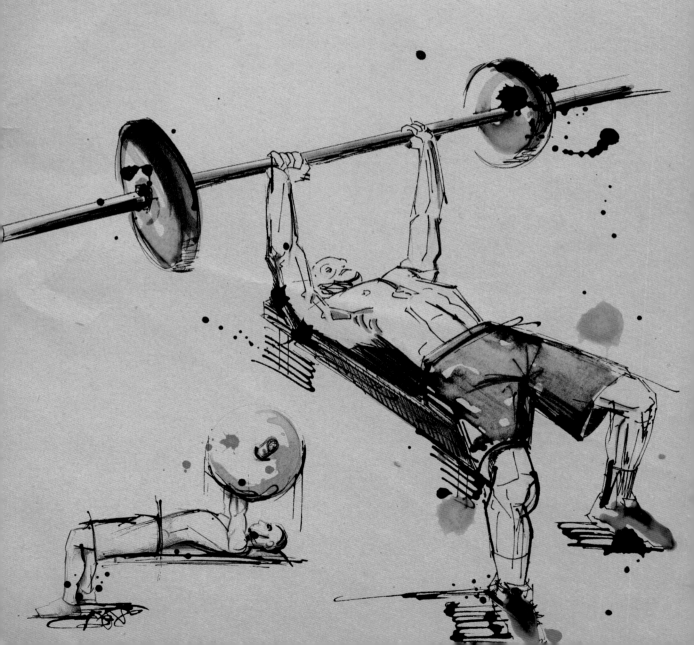

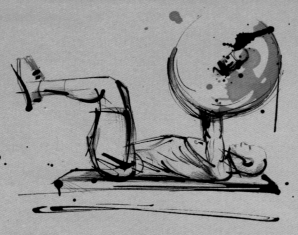 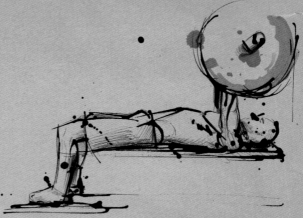

Technique tips

- Foot placement: traditionally spread wide with feet flat on the floor (but this can be modified).

- Back placement: As primary support for pushing the bar up, the back (and especially the shoulder blades) is solidly anchored to the bench with the spinal column perfectly centered. Try to keep the shoulder blades as close to each other as possible.

- Head placement: firmly on the bench with the chin lowered and the neck flexed to its natural position.

- Hand grip on the bar: The bar should be locked in place with the thumbs. The traditional grip is wider than shoulder-width, but it can also be wider or narrower. For maximum anatomical comfort, we recommend a shoulder-width grip.

- Elbow position: Keep the elbows in line with the shoulders.

- Starting position for the bar: After removing the bar from the rack, hold it above your chest with straight arms.

- Lowering the bar: With constant control, lower the bar just to the base of your chest. Touch your torso without resting the weight or bouncing the bar off your torso and then immediately start to push the bar back up.

- Pushing the bar up: This movement should be as explosive as possible to overcome gravity. The trajectory of the bar is not in a straight line, but slightly curved toward the rack.

- Stabilizing the bar: Stabilize the bar at the end of each rep with the elbows fully extended, above the chest. Momentarily hold the bar after the last rep before placing it on the rack.

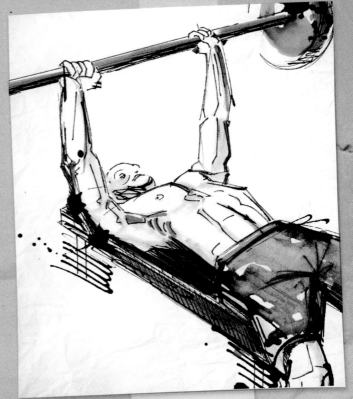

→ Read more about shoulder impingements on page 72.

WORKOUT - BENCH PRESSES

WORKOUT 1 - PULL BEFORE PUSHING

10 X 1 DEADLIFTS (PAGE 125) AT 85 TO 90 PERCENT OF MAXIMUM, STARTING EVERY MINUTE

THEN, AS MANY TIMES AS POSSIBLE IN 8 MINUTES: 7 BENCH PRESSES, 9 BURPEES (PAGE 165), AND 12 KETTLEBELL SWINGS (PAGE 128)

WORKOUT 2 - DRIVE THRESHOLD

4 X 8 SQUATS (PAGE 89) AT 80 PERCENT OF MAXIMUM IN LESS THAN 10 MINUTES

THEN, AS MANY TIMES AS POSSIBLE IN 10 MINUTES: 10 PULL-UPS (PAGE 143), 10 BENCH PRESSES AT 60 PERCENT OF MAXIMUM, AND 200-METER SPRINT

WORKOUT 3 - PURE STRENGTH

10 X 2 SQUATS (PAGE 89), TRYING TO INCREASE THE WEIGHT EACH SET

10 X 2 BENCH PRESSES, TRYING TO INCREASE THE WEIGHT EACH SET

BENCH PRESS WITH DUMBBELLS OR KETTLEBELLS

The most well-known version of this exercise is done with dumbbells or kettlebells, and its primary limitation is using an average amount of weight. When workouts involve heavier weights, you may not have the appropriate weights or you may have trouble organizing them without a rack (some rack models are available). But working with dumbbells and kettlebells is good for long workouts and allows you to balance the work for both arms.

You may also alternate arms, either by lifting one and then the other (the weights pass each other at the beginning and end of the movement so that only one weight moves at a time) or by alternating one and then the other (the weights pass each other in the middle of the movement so that both weights move at the same time).

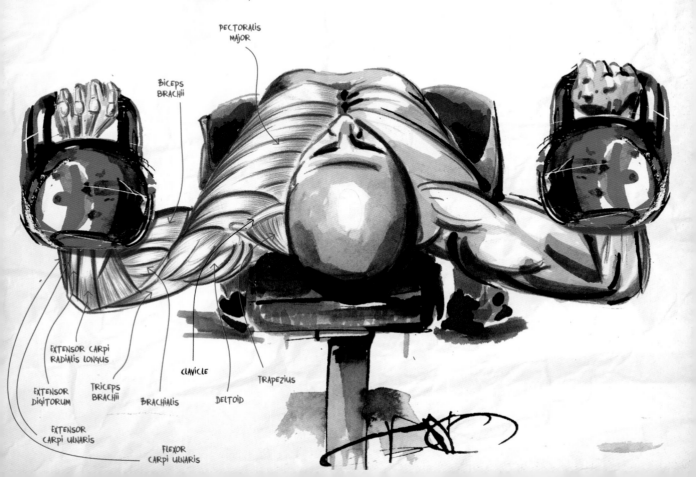

PECTORALIS MAJOR

BICEPS BRACHII

EXTENSOR CARPI RADIALIS LONGUS

EXTENSOR DIGITORUM

TRICEPS BRACHII

BRACHIALIS

CLAVICLE

DELTOID

TRAPEZIUS

EXTENSOR CARPI ULNARIS

FLEXOR CARPI ULNARIS

WORKOUT – BENCH PRESSES WITH DUMBBELLS OR KETTLEBELLS

WORKOUT 1 – SNEAKY PUSH

4 X 8 BENCH PRESSES AT 80 PERCENT OF MAXIMUM, RECOVERY 90 SECONDS
THEN, EVERY MINUTE FOR 12 MINUTES:
8 BENCH PRESSES WITH DUMBBELLS/KETTLEBELLS

WORKOUT 2 – INFINITE PUSH

AS MANY TIMES AS POSSIBLE IN 20 MINUTES:
25 SIT-UPS, 21 BENCH
PRESSES WITH DUMBBELLS/
KETTLEBELLS, 400-METER RUN

WORKOUT 3 – SQUAT RECOVERY

5 ROUNDS: 10 BENCH PRESSES AT 75 PERCENT OF MAXIMUM, 5 CLAPPING PUSH-UPS (PAGE 167), 10 SQUATS (PAGE 89) AT 60 PERCENT OF MAXIMUM, 10 KNEE TUCK JUMPS, 10 BENCH PRESSES AT 50 PERCENT OF MAXIMUM, 5 PUSH-UPS (PAGE 158). RECOVERY: 90 SECONDS

Using a ball instead of a bench

Another version that is used more often today replaces the bench with a stability ball. That version is mainly preventive, so we are excluding it from our programs. When you are on the path to developing strength, requiring the body to stay in balance during an exercise is less effective than using a stable bench. Also, given the extreme fatigue that occurs in high intensity training— and the loss of focus that may go along with it—we prefer training situations that are stable and secure.

✖ DEADLIFT

This exercise involves lifting a bar off the ground and bringing it to the front of the thighs or hips with the body standing tall and the arms straight. The muscles that are primarily recruited during a deadlift are the quadriceps (rectus femoris, vastus lateralis, vastus medialis, and crural fascia), the buttocks (gluteus minimus, medius, and maximus as well as fasciae latae and the tensor fasciae latae), and the lumbar muscles. The bar is held with straight arms; therefore, the forearms, shoulders, and trapezius muscles are also involved. The hamstrings (semitendinosus, semimembranosus, and biceps femoris) support the pelvis, and the gastrocnemius and soleus stabilize the calves.

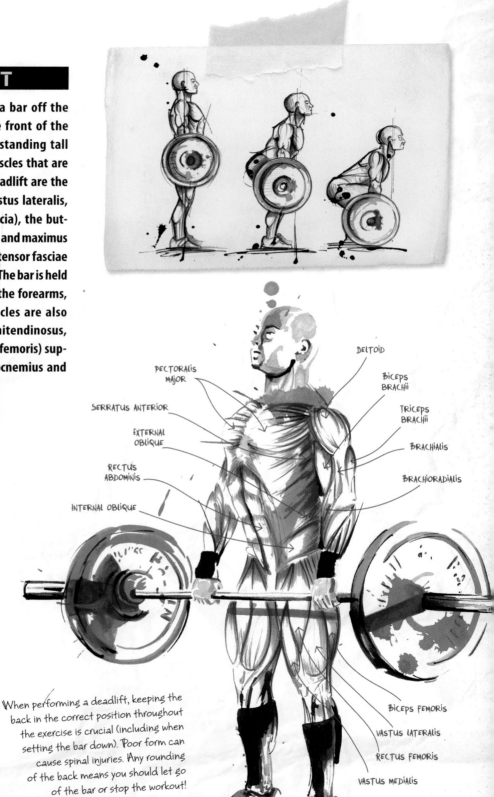

Avoid this!

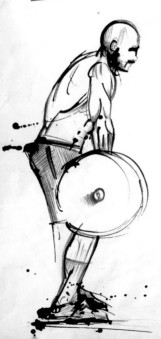

PECTORALIS MAJOR

SERRATUS ANTERIOR

EXTERNAL OBLIQUE

RECTUS ABDOMINIS

INTERNAL OBLIQUE

DELTOID

BICEPS BRACHII

TRICEPS BRACHII

BRACHIALIS

BRACHIORADIALIS

BICEPS FEMORIS

VASTUS LATERALIS

RECTUS FEMORIS

VASTUS MEDIALIS

When performing a deadlift, keeping the back in the correct position throughout the exercise is crucial (including when setting the bar down). Poor form can cause spinal injuries. Any rounding of the back means you should let go of the bar or stop the workout!

Technique tips

In the starting position, your feet should be hip-width apart and your hips should be in the same plane as your knees (higher or lower depending on body dimensions). Your torso should be as straight as possible from the beginning to the end of the movement to reduce stress on the lower back. The feet are in line with the femurs. The back is straight and leaning forward, but it should never be rounded. The synergistic muscle action of the quadriceps, back muscles, buttocks, and hamstrings is the most important point.

- Weight placement: The feet should be perfectly flat on the floor, and the body weight should be distributed evenly over the entire foot. When possible, wear shoes with thin, stiff soles.

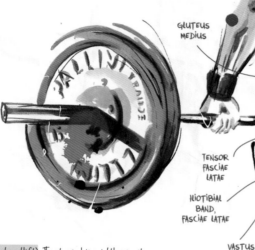

- Stance (traditional deadlift): Feet are hip-width apart.

- Stance (sumo deadlift): Feet are wider than hip- or shoulder-width apart.

- Hand placement and grip: Use a pronated or mixed grip, with the hands shoulder-width apart.

- Back position: Control the forward tilt of the pelvis and hold the back straight throughout the exercise.

- Starting position: The shoulders are pulled back, the chest is sticking out, the hips are in almost the same plane as the knees, and the pelvis tilted forward with control.

- Head position: The gaze should be fixed on a point directly in front.

- The deadlift: Put the arms under tension and stand up with your back straight. The bar brushes along the legs until you are upright and balanced.

- Prepare for the descent: Follow the reverse path but do not release control of your back.

- Critical moments: The first is below the knees, and the other is just after the knees. In both cases, you risk losing control of the back. For that reason, your form has to be better than ever.

- Breathing: Breathe in while in the starting position as you place tension on your muscles. Stand up without breathing and then exhale after you reach the final position.

Muscle labels (figure): TRAPEZIUS · TERES MINOR · TERES MAJOR · INFRASPINATUS · LATISSIMUS DORSI · EXTERNAL OBLIQUE · GLUTEUS MAXIMUS · GLUTEUS MEDIUS · TENSOR FASCIAE LATAE · ILIOTIBIAL BAND, FASCIAE LATAE · VASTUS LATERALIS · ADDUCTOR MAGNUS · GRACILIS · SEMITENDINOSUS · BICEPS FEMORIS

Remember that whole-body exercises involving the lower body (deadlifts and squats) isolate the agonist muscles from the antagonist muscles much less than whole-body exercises involving the upper body (bench press or pull-ups). Tests that we have conducted with electromyography (EMG) show, for most athletes, differences of only 10 to 20 percent between the quadriceps and the hamstrings!

WORKOUT - DEADLIFTS

WORKOUT 1 - STANDING ON THE HORIZON

AS FAST AS POSSIBLE: 10 X 15 DEADLIFTS,
15 PUSH-UPS (PAGE 158), MAX RECOVERY
AFTER THE PUSH-UPS: 1 MINUTE

ADD-ON CIRCUIT: 5 X 8 BARBELL AB ROLLOUTS
(PAGE 191), 20-SECOND HANDSTAND

WORKOUT 2 - POWER DEADLIFTS

4 X 5 MAX DEADLIFTS FOLLOWED BY 20-METER RUN

THEN 3 ROUNDS: 3 DEADLIFTS, 10 SIT-UPS,
15 BURPEES (PAGE 165)

WORKOUT 3 - AEROBIC DEADLIFTS

10 ROUNDS: 5 DEADLIFTS AT YOUR 5-REP MAX,
600-METER LOW INTENSITY RUN

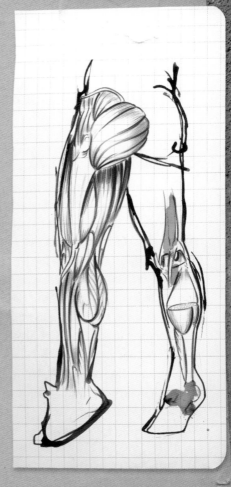

SPECIAL CONCERN: VULNERABLE HAMSTRINGS

THE HAMSTRINGS ARE ESPECIALLY VULNERABLE MUSCLES WITH MULTIPLE ATTACHMENTS. THEY ARE OFTEN
UNDERDEVELOPED EVEN THOUGH THEY BEAR A LOT OF WEIGHT ECCENTRICALLY. AS YOU PREPARE FOR A
WORKOUT, YOU SHOULD PAY CLOSE ATTENTION TO BALANCING THE WORK WITH THEIR ANTAGONIST MUSCLES,
THE QUADRICEPS. THEREFORE, YOU SHOULD CONSCIENTIOUSLY WARM UP THE HAMSTRINGS.

WHEN A WORKOUT INCLUDES A LOT OF HAMSTRING WORK, WE RECOMMEND THAT YOU DO KNEE RAISES
AT VARYING HEIGHTS, FORWARD OR BACKWARD RUNNING WITH GRADUALLY INCREASING SPEED, OR EVEN
GRADUALLY INCREASING TENSION USING SMALL BRIDGES OR CONTRACTION/RELAXATION MOVEMENTS.

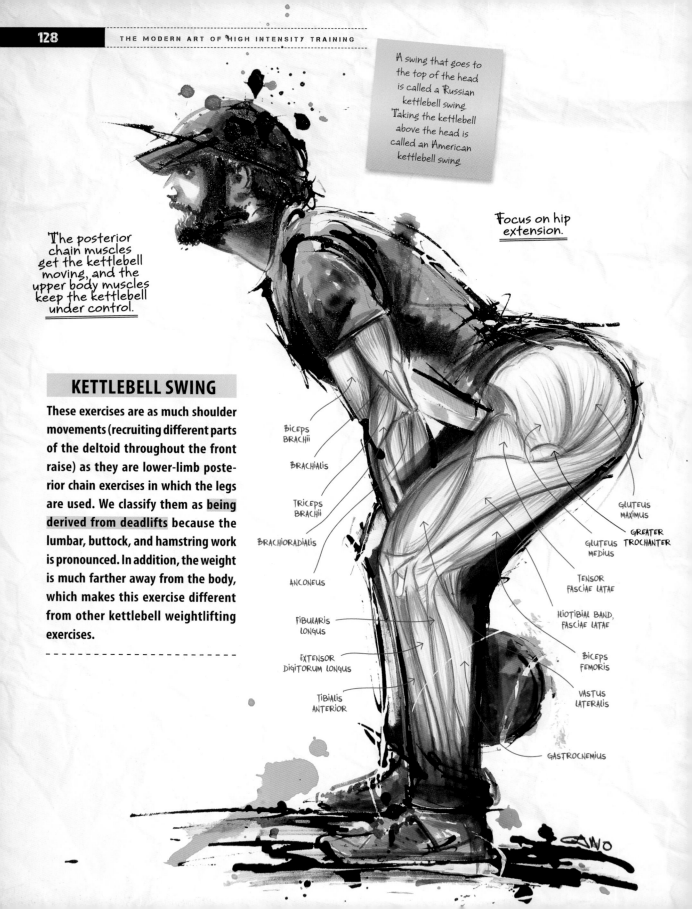

A swing that goes to the top of the head is called a Russian kettlebell swing. Taking the kettlebell above the head is called an American kettlebell swing.

Focus on hip extension.

The posterior chain muscles get the kettlebell moving, and the upper body muscles keep the kettlebell under control.

KETTLEBELL SWING

These exercises are as much shoulder movements (recruiting different parts of the deltoid throughout the front raise) as they are lower-limb posterior chain exercises in which the legs are used. We classify them as **being derived from deadlifts** because the lumbar, buttock, and hamstring work is pronounced. In addition, the weight is much farther away from the body, which makes this exercise different from other kettlebell weightlifting exercises.

BICEPS BRACHII

BRACHIALIS

TRICEPS BRACHII

BRACHIORADIALIS

ANCONEUS

FIBULARIS LONGUS

EXTENSOR DIGITORUM LONGUS

TIBIALIS ANTERIOR

GLUTEUS MAXIMUS

GREATER TROCHANTER

GLUTEUS MEDIUS

TENSOR FASCIAE LATAE

ILIOTIBIAL BAND, FASCIAE LATAE

BICEPS FEMORIS

VASTUS LATERALIS

GASTROCNEMIUS

Kettlebell swing methods

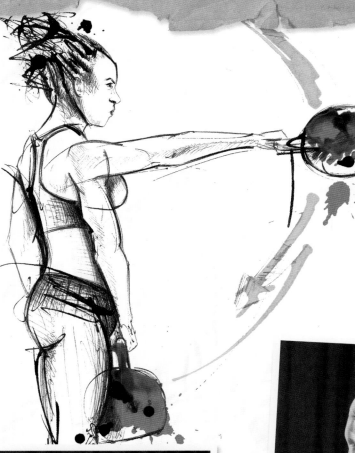

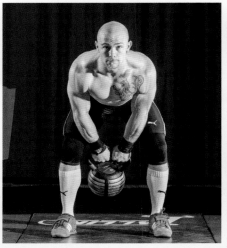

Two-handed grip

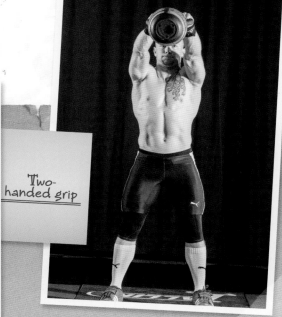

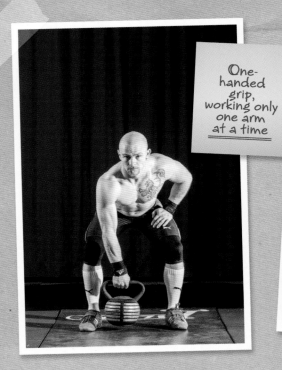

One-handed grip, working only one arm at a time

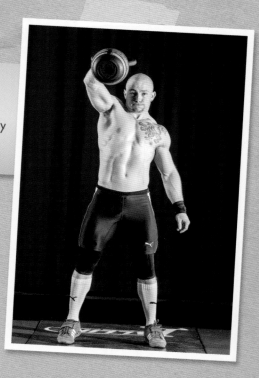

One-handed grip, changing hands at the bottom of the rep

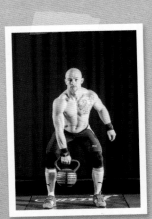

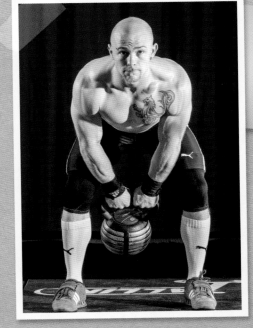

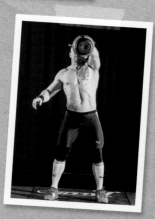

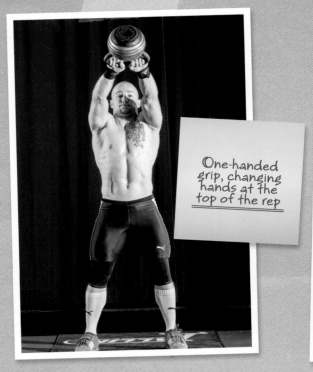

One-handed grip, changing hands at the top of the rep

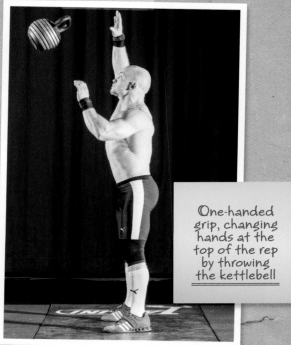

One-handed grip, changing hands at the top of the rep by throwing the kettlebell

There are two versions for one or two hands:

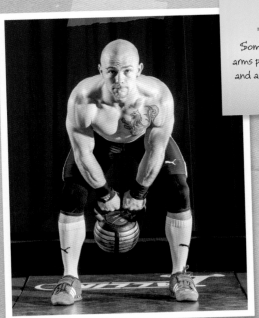

Height

Somewhere between arms parallel to the floor and arms perpendicular to the floor

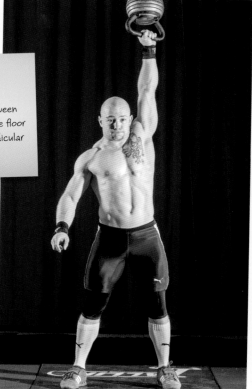

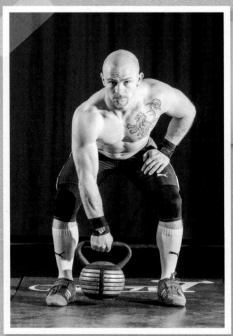

The kettlebell can be placed on the floor every rep or not.

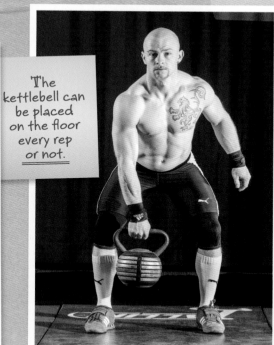

Note

You can also use the legs for assistance to a greater or lesser degree by doing a single or double "wave" and bending the knees (a little or a lot) before and after each hip bend.

Technique tips

Holding the kettlebell or kettlebells in a pronated grip, flex the hips and knees slightly and lean forward with your back straight and your pelvis tilted forward to get the kettlebells moving. Pull your shoulders back with your arms straight before beginning the upward movement. Extend your hips and knees to stand up as you lift the kettlebell. You should be standing as your arms reach a level where they are parallel to the floor. When you are standing, the knees and hips should be fully extended, the abdominal muscles and buttocks should be contracted, the head should be straight, and the gaze should be fixed on a point slightly above the horizon.

WORKOUT – KETTLEBELL SWINGS

WORKOUT 1 – TEA TIME

AS MANY ROUNDS AS POSSIBLE IN 12 MINUTES:

20 FULL PULL-UPS WITH A BAND (PAGE 143),
20 ONE-HANDED KETTLEBELL SWINGS, 200-METER RUN

THEN 5 ROUNDS OF 3 MINUTES WITH 1 MINUTE OF ACTIVE REST

ADD-ON WORKOUT: 1.8-MILE (3 KM) RUN AT 50 PERCENT OF MAX INTENSITY

WORKOUT 2 – KETTLE RUN

10-MINUTE RUN AT 60 PERCENT OF MAX INTENSITY

QUICK RUN: 800 METERS

100 TWO-HANDED KETTLEBELL SWINGS (RECOVERY: YOUR CHOICE)

QUICK RUN: 800 METERS

100 ONE-HANDED KETTLEBELL SWINGS (RECOVERY: YOUR CHOICE)

QUICK RUN: 800 METERS

3 SETS OF PULL-UPS (PAGE 143), AS MANY REPS AS POSSIBLE

WORKOUT 3 – FROM RUSSIA WITH LOVE

5 SETS, 1 MINUTE EACH, AS MANY ROUNDS AS POSSIBLE:
4 TWO-HANDED KETTLEBELL SWINGS AND 180-DEGREE ROTATION, 2 KETTLEBELL
GOBLET SQUATS (PAGE 98). RECOVERY BETWEEN SETS: 1 MINUTE

10 SETS OF 100-METER SHUTTLE RUN, 10 BURPEES (PAGE 165),
10 ALTERNATING KETTLEBELL SWINGS, 1 MINUTE OF RECOVERY BETWEEN
SETS. 3 MINUTES OF RECOVERY BETWEEN SETS 5 AND 6

ARABESQUE

This powerful and difficult exercise strengthens the posterior chain and is really just a one-leg deadlift. It can be done with a bar, two kettlebells or dumbbells, or a single kettlebell or dumbbell working one side at a time. Throughout the exercise, the back and the free leg must be in perfect alignment. The hips should be fully open (do not collapse the body). Finally, be careful not to twist the torso; the chest should always face forward.

Arm-leg opposition, see photos →

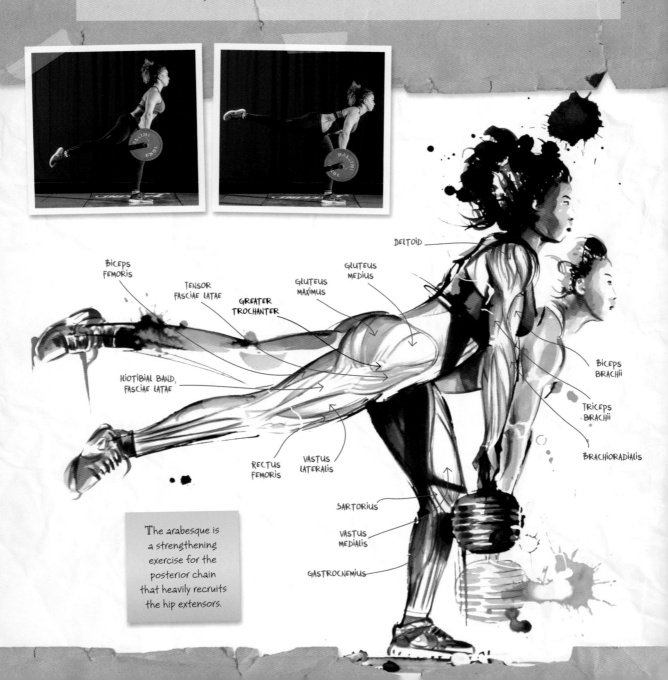

DELTOID

GLUTEUS MEDIUS

GLUTEUS MAXIMUS

BICEPS FEMORIS

TENSOR FASCIAE LATAE

GREATER TROCHANTER

ILIOTIBIAL BAND, FASCIAE LATAE

RECTUS FEMORIS

VASTUS LATERALIS

SARTORIUS

VASTUS MEDIALIS

GASTROCNEMIUS

BICEPS BRACHII

TRICEPS BRACHII

BRACHIORADIALIS

The arabesque is a strengthening exercise for the posterior chain that heavily recruits the hip extensors.

WORKOUT - ARABESQUES

WORKOUT 1 - SWAN LAKE

SQUAT (PAGE 89) COUNTDOWN (INCREASING WEIGHT):
5, 4, 3, 2, 1 IN LESS THAN 15 MINUTES

5 ROUNDS: 20 ARABESQUES WITH ALTERNATING DUMBBELLS,
15 PUSH-UPS (PAGE 158), 20 ALTERNATING LUNGES HOLDING
A KETTLEBELL (PAGE 140), 10 PULL-UPS (PAGE 143)

RECOVERY: 2 MINUTES

WORKOUT 2 - COMPLEX DEADLIFTS

10 ROUNDS: 1 HEAVY DEADLIFT (PAGE 125), 1 ARABESQUE
PER LEG, 1 HEAVY DEADLIFT, 1 ARABESQUE PER LEG

RECOVERY: 2 TO 3 MINUTES

WORKOUT 3 - LONG WINTER'S NIGHT

AS MANY TIMES AS POSSIBLE IN 17 MINUTES:
10 ARABESQUES (RIGHT LEG), 100 ABDOMINAL EXERCISES (VARIED),
10 ARABESQUES (LEFT LEG), 10 PUSH-UPS (PAGE 158),
100 ABDOMINAL EXERCISES (VARIED)

STRAIGHT-LEG DEADLIFT

This version, as the name indicates, involves limiting the bend in the knees to train the erector spinae to a greater degree. Be careful not to round the back or let the pelvis tilt backward, an error commonly seen in this style of exercise (see the section on disc injures on page 58 to understand the risks better).

Keep the chest open and the shoulders pulled back.

WORKOUT – STRAIGHT-LEG DEADLIFTS

WORKOUT 1 – SEMISTRAIGHT

5 X 10 STRAIGHT-LEG DEADLIFTS

5 X 5 DEADLIFTS (PAGE 125)

THEN AS MANY TIMES AS POSSIBLE IN 10 MINUTES:
2 STRAIGHT-LEG DEADLIFTS AT 50 TO 60 PERCENT OF MAXIMUM,
3 DEADLIFTS WITHOUT CHANGING THE WEIGHT,
10 BENCH PRESSES WITH DUMBBELLS/KETTLEBELLS

WORKOUT 2 – MADLACK

5 SETS OF 3 CLEANS (PAGE 34) AND 4 KNEE TUCK JUMPS

THEN, TAKING AS MUCH RECOVERY TIME AS WORKING
TIME, 6 X 20 STRAIGHT-LEG DEADLIFTS

WORKOUT 3 – COLOMBIANA

5 X 5 SQUATS (PAGE 89)

EVERY MINUTE FOR 15 MINUTES:
1 STRAIGHT-LEG DEADLIFT AT 80 PERCENT OF MAXIMUM,
1 SQUAT AT 70 PERCENT OF MAXIMUM, 1 HIGH BOX JUMP

SUMO DEADLIFT

Well known among power lifters, this exercise is a good alternative to the traditional deadlift for those who want to lift heavy weights. It does not recruit the posterior chain in the same way, so we recommend varying the use of these lifts in your workout. The same basic principles apply, but you use a slightly narrower grip and keep the feet in a wider stance (wider than hip- or shoulder-width apart). More than ever, you need to keep the chest open and the shoulders pulled back to avoid a risky kyphosis. A sumo deadlift is often combined with a high pull.

WORKOUT – SUMO DEADLIFTS

WORKOUT 1 – THE 3 15

3 X 5 DEADLIFTS (PAGE 125)

3 TO 5 ROUNDS AS FAST AS POSSIBLE: 15 PULL-UPS (PAGE 143), 15 BURPEES (PUSH-UP AND KNEE-TUCK JUMP, PAGE 165), 15 SUMO DEADLIFTS

WORKOUT 2 – MAKISUSHI

AS FAST AS POSSIBLE:

15 SUMO DEADLIFTS, 30 PULL-UPS

12 SUMO DEADLIFTS, 25 PULL-UPS

10 SUMO DEADLIFTS, 20 PULL-UPS

8 SUMO DEADLIFTS, 15 PULL-UPS

6 SUMO DEADLIFTS, 10 PULL-UPS

5 SUMO DEADLIFTS, 5 PULL-UPS

WORKOUT 3 – SAKURA

3 X 5 SQUATS (PAGE 89)

AS FAST AS POSSIBLE: 21, 18, 15, 12, 9, 6, 3 REPS OF SUMO DEADLIFTS ALTERNATED WITH SHOULDER PRESSES

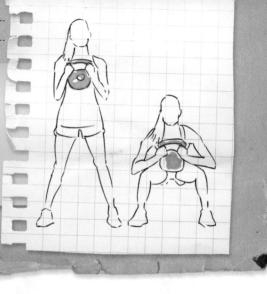

LUNGE

This exercise comes in many versions: bar on the shoulder or above the head (snatch lunge), with dumbbells held in straight arms, with a kettlebell held against the chest, and others. The lunge itself can also be done to the front, to the back, or to the side. The athlete can then come back to the starting position, called a lunge in place. The athlete can also keep the feet stationary; the feet remain in the lunge position while the body is lowered and raised. This is a split squat. Finally, the athlete can move in marching lunges, which is simply walking in a lunge. The athlete can also focus on tiring out one leg before switching sides, or she or he can switch legs on every rep. Some workouts may include a jumping version of lunges in which the front and back legs switch in the air during a jump. Lunges recruit the quadriceps, biceps femoris, and glutes. A longer step works the glutes more, whereas a shorter step works the quadriceps more.

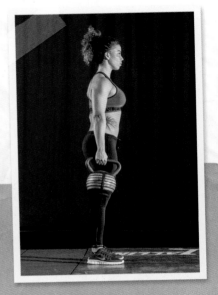

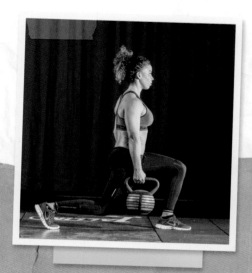

Technique tips

In the starting position, the feet are parallel and slightly less than hip-width apart. If you are doing a forward lunge with a bar, then the bar should be on the back of your shoulders—never on your neck—to reduce the pressure on your spine. If you are doing a forward lunge with dumbbells, then hold the dumbbells with your arms straight at your sides. If you are doing the lunge with kettlebells, you can hold them at your sides as you would the dumbbells or just hold one against your chest with your arms bent. Be careful not to let the weight of the kettlebell pull you forward and cause you to round your back or lean forward. Keep your knees and feet parallel (do not open the back foot as in a fencing lunge), take a large step forward, and then bend the forward leg until the knee of your back leg brushes the ground. Return to the starting position by pushing with your forward leg. If you are doing marching lunges, the forward leg supports your weight as you stand up and bring the back leg forward next to the front leg.

Adjust your lunges depending on your goals.

Jumping lunges to help increase your power

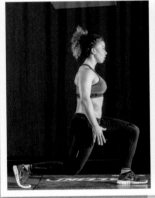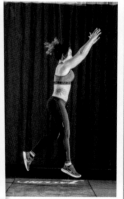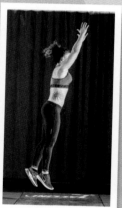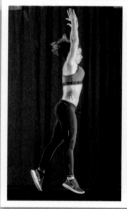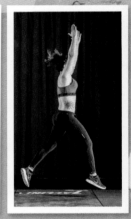

Snatch lunges for overall body stability

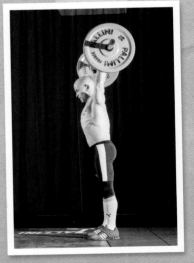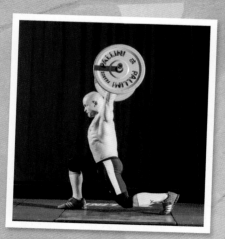

WORKOUT - LUNGES

WORKOUT 1 - LUNGE FANTASY

5 ROUNDS: 50 ALTERNATING LUNGES, 21 BURPEES (PAGE 165)

WORKOUT 2 - KILIMANJARO

30 ALTERNATING LUNGES AT 40 PERCENT OF MAXIMUM,
21 PULL-UPS (PAGE 143), 21 SIT-UPS

28 ALTERNATING LUNGES, 18 PULL-UPS, 18 SIT-UPS

26 ALTERNATING LUNGES, 16 PULL-UPS, 16 SIT-UPS

24 ALTERNATING LUNGES, 14 PULL-UPS, 14 SIT-UPS

22 ALTERNATING LUNGES, 12 PULL-UPS, 12 SIT-UPS

20 ALTERNATING LUNGES, 10 PULL-UPS, 10 SIT-UPS

18 ALTERNATING LUNGES, 8 PULL-UPS, 8 SIT-UPS

16 ALTERNATING LUNGES, 6 PULL-UPS, 6 SIT-UPS

WORKOUT 3 - LUNGE POWER

3 X 3 SNATCHES (PAGE 60)

3 X 5 SQUATS (PAGE 89)

3 TIMES AS FAST AS POSSIBLE: 3 SNATCHES, 30 METERS
OF MARCHING LUNGES, 20 BURPEES (PAGE 165)

BODYWEIGHT EXERCISES

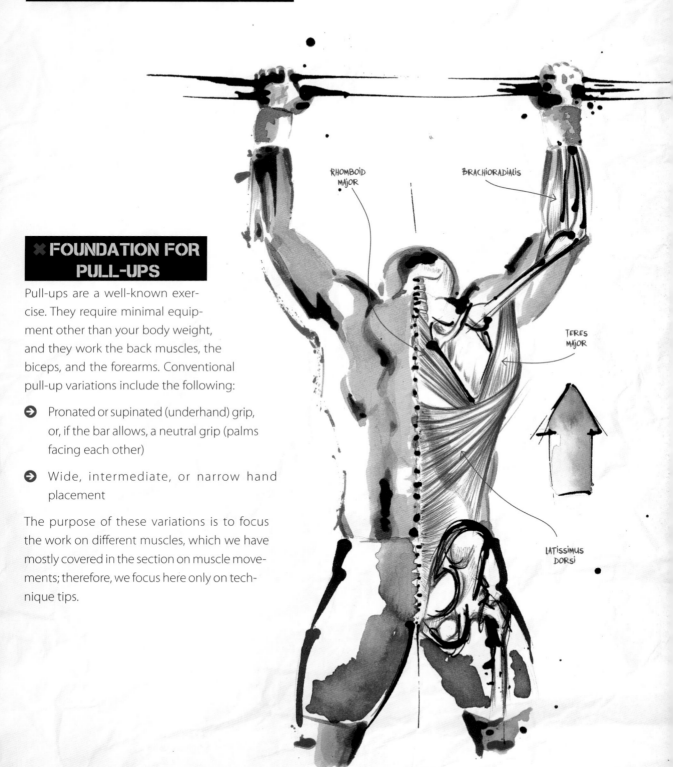

RHOMBOID MAJOR

BRACHIORADIALIS

TERES MAJOR

LATISSIMUS DORSI

✖ FOUNDATION FOR PULL-UPS

Pull-ups are a well-known exercise. They require minimal equipment other than your body weight, and they work the back muscles, the biceps, and the forearms. Conventional pull-up variations include the following:

➡ Pronated or supinated (underhand) grip, or, if the bar allows, a neutral grip (palms facing each other)

➡ Wide, intermediate, or narrow hand placement

The purpose of these variations is to focus the work on different muscles, which we have mostly covered in the section on muscle movements; therefore, we focus here only on technique tips.

Technique tips

Grab the bar, squeeze your
shoulder blades together without
exaggerating the lumbar curve,
and pull your body straight up.
You can stretch your arms out
(see the drawing) but do not let
yourself fall with straight arms
without slowing yourself down
because the shock could cause
joint instability. Finally, as with any
pulling exercise, focus on pulling
your shoulder blades together
at the beginning of the exercise
to increase the tension in the
back as well as to improve your
shoulder control (see page 86).

RADIUS

TRAPEZIUS

ULNA

HUMERUS

SCAPULAE

TERES MAJOR

LATISSIMUS DORSI

INTERNAL
OBLIQUE

RIB

GLUTEUS
MEDIUS

GLUTEUS
MAXIMUS

HIP BONE

HEAD OF THE FEMUR

FASCIAE
LATAE

FEMUR

BICEPS FEMORIS

VASTUS LATERALIS

SEMIMEMBRANOSUS

ADDUCTOR
LONGUS

The danger is not
in allowing the
arms to straighten,
but in letting the
body fall suddenly.
Even when working
at a fast speed,
you must control
your descent.

WORKOUT - PULL-UPS

WORKOUT 1 - ARMS AND LEGS

5 ROUNDS: AS MANY REPS AS POSSIBLE OF FRONT SQUATS (PAGE 97) AND THEN PULL-UPS

WORKOUT 2 - CAPITAL

3 ROUNDS:

100-METER RUN

12 PULL-UPS

100-METER RUN

24 ALTERNATING KETTLEBELL SWINGS (PAGE 130)

200-METER RUN

WORKOUT 3 - TIRE AND SQUAT

3 ROUNDS: 21, 15, 9 REPS IN SQUATS (PAGE 89) AND THEN PULL-UPS

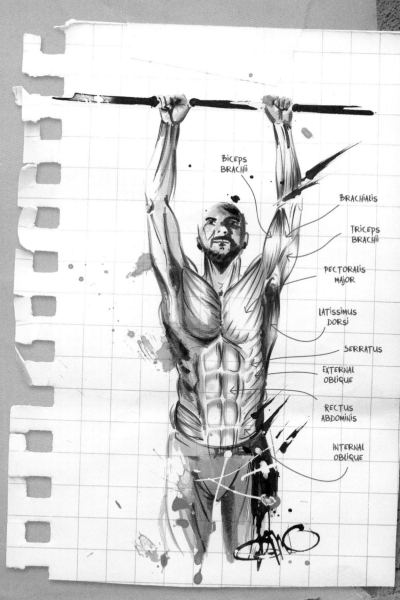

BICEPS BRACHII

BRACHIALIS

TRICEPS BRACHII

PECTORALIS MAJOR

LATISSIMUS DORSI

SERRATUS

EXTERNAL OBLIQUE

RECTUS ABDOMINIS

INTERNAL OBLIQUE

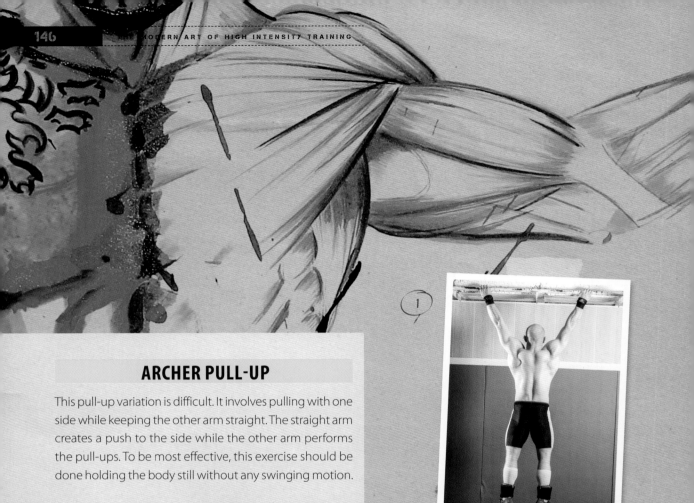

ARCHER PULL-UP

This pull-up variation is difficult. It involves pulling with one side while keeping the other arm straight. The straight arm creates a push to the side while the other arm performs the pull-ups. To be most effective, this exercise should be done holding the body still without any swinging motion.

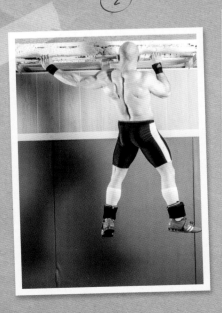

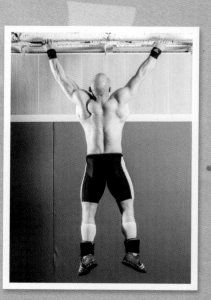

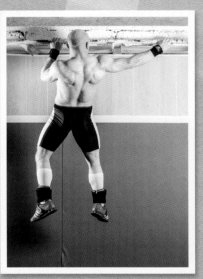

WORKOUT – ARCHER PULL-UPS

WORKOUT 1 – THE 4 x 100

CHOOSE THE NUMBER OF SETS YOU WANT TO DO FOR THESE REPS:

100 ARCHER PULL-UPS

100 AIR SQUATS

100 CLAPPING PUSH-UPS (PAGE 167)

100 BOX JUMPS

WORKOUT 2 – SANDS OF DEATH

EVERY MINUTE: 10 REGULAR PULL-UPS (PAGE 143), 10 ARCHER PULL-UPS, 10 CLAPPING PULL-UPS (PAGE 148), 10 REGULAR PULL-UPS, 10 ARCHER PULL-UPS, 10 CLAPPING PULL-UPS, 10 REGULAR PULL-UPS

5-KILOMETER RUN

WORKOUT 3 – BRITISH ARCHER

5 ROUNDS, NO TIME LIMIT, WITH 3 MINUTES OF ACTIVE RECOVERY BETWEEN ROUNDS: 3 CLEANS (PAGE 34), 10 ARCHER PULL-UPS, 6 BOX JUMPS, 10 ARCHER PULL-UPS, 5 SQUATS (PAGE 89), 10 ARCHER PULL-UPS, 3 CLEANS

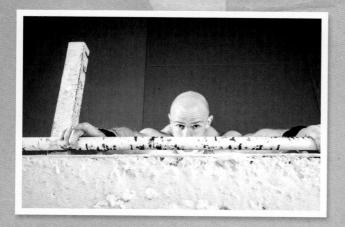

OPEN-HAND (CLAPPING) PULL-UP

This exercise is the same as the basic version of a pull-up, but you should generate as much power as you can during the concentric phase of the movement so that you will be able to open your hands (and perhaps even clap them) as your chin passes the bar. During this exercise, pay close attention to the descent, which is often fast. Slow yourself down enough to limit the impact on your joints at the end of the movement.

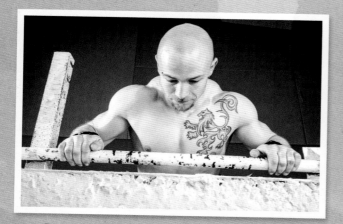

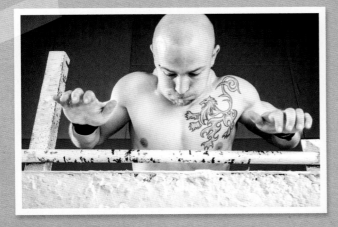

You will need time to gain confidence, learn the rhythm of the exercise, and judge the proper time to <u>let go of the bar.</u>

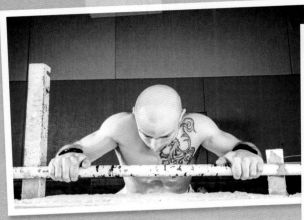

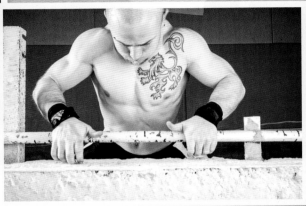

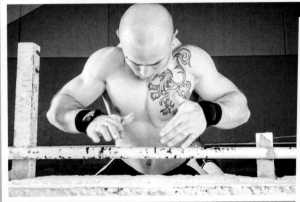

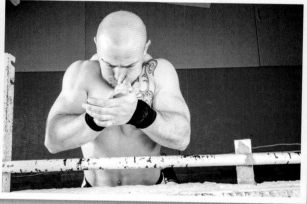

The clapping pull-up is an explosive exercise better suited for short sets (fewer than 8 reps) than for long sets.

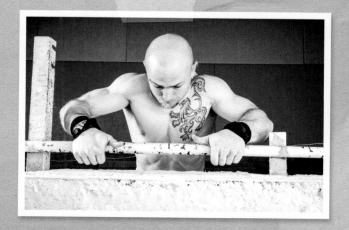

WORKOUT – CLAPPING PULL-UPS

WORKOUT 1 – CLAP, CLAP, CLAP

3 X 3 SNATCHES (PAGE 60)

3 X 5 OVERHEAD SQUATS (PAGE 100)

AS MANY TIMES AS POSSIBLE IN 12 MINUTES: 4 CLAPPING PULL-UPS, 6 CLAPPING PUSH-UPS (PAGE 167), 10 KNEE TUCK JUMPS (MINIMUM CONTACT TIME WITH THE GROUND, MAXIMUM HEIGHT)

WORKOUT 2 – POWER CLAP

5 X 5 SQUATS (PAGE 89)

6 ROUNDS, 2 TO 3 MINUTES OF REST BETWEEN ROUNDS: 3 SNATCHES (PAGE 60), 6 MAX VERTICAL JUMPS, 6 CLAPPING PULL-UPS

WORKOUT 3 – THE END OF TIME

3 X 5 BENCH PRESSES (PAGE 121)

3 X 5 DEADLIFTS (PAGE 125)

6 ROUNDS, 2 MINUTES OF RECOVERY BETWEEN ROUNDS: 3 CLEAN AND JERKS (PAGE 34) AT 70 PERCENT OF MAXIMUM, 4 CLAPPING PULL-UPS, 10 PUSH-UPS (PAGE 158), 10 AIR SQUATS AND KNEE TUCK JUMPS

Assisted Pull-Ups

A weak point of some high intensity training programs is that beginners, who are not yet strong enough, attempt to complete workouts that are above their fitness level. As a result, they are exposed to high risk of injury, which happens most often in bodyweight exercises. As an example, a young man who weighs 187 pounds (85 kg). A simple pull-up represents a weight likely far above his maximum for 1 rep. You would not ask him to pull 187 pounds (85 kg) on a pulley weight. Therefore, being able to adjust the body weight is crucial. Assistance from a partner or the use of an elastic band can help the athlete reduce the bodyweight load.

An assisted pull-up is also great for experienced athletes working in long sets. Anticipating a loss of technique and facilitating the task in advance is better than cheating on the movement after you get tired.

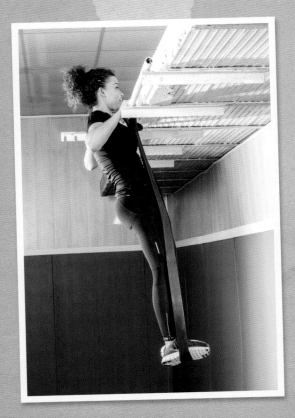

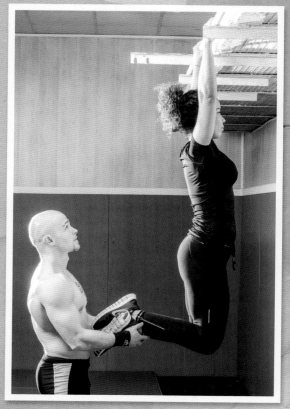

Muscle-up

In contrast to an assisted pull-up, this type of pull-up is far more difficult. Using the initial momentum and a light swing, bring your shoulders above the bar and engage your arms to push up until your arms are completely straight.

How to do a muscle-up in four steps:

1. Strengthen the pulling muscles through a variety of pull-ups.

2. Practice the swing by pulling explosively with the goal of pulling the shoulders above the bar.

3. Practice the complete movement while using multiple resistance bands to provide assistance.

4. Over time, gradually remove the bands until you can lift your full body weight.

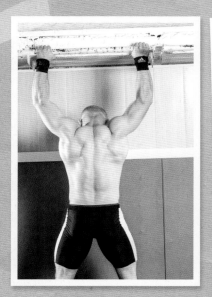
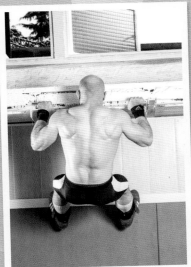
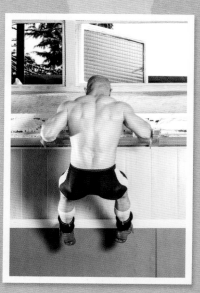

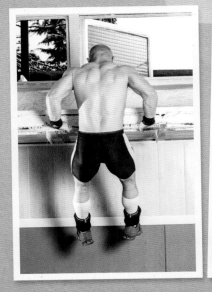
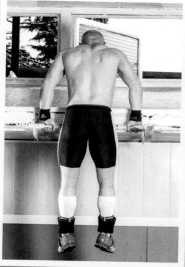
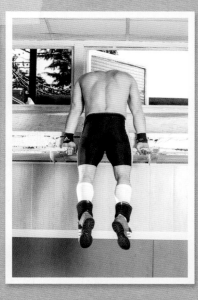

WORKOUT - PULL-UPS

WORKOUT 1 - NINJA GAIDEN

3 X 3 SNATCHES (PAGE 60)

3 X 5 OVERHEAD SQUATS (PAGE 100)

5 ROUNDS WITH 3 MINUTES OF RECOVERY BETWEEN ROUNDS:

1 TO 3 PULL-UPS (AT YOUR LEVEL), 3 SQUATS (PAGE 89), 50-METER SPRINT

WORKOUT 2 - BALKAN GYMNAST

10 X 1 SQUATS (PAGE 89) WITH 1 MINUTE OF RECOVERY MAX

5 ROUNDS WITH 2 MINUTES REST OF BETWEEN ROUNDS FOR PERFECT TECHNIQUE (LOSS OF FORM MEANS YOU STOP THE EXERCISE IMMEDIATELY): AS MANY NEUTRAL GRIP PULL-UPS AS POSSIBLE, AS MANY PRONATED GRIP PULL-UPS AS POSSIBLE, AS MANY SUPINATED GRIP PULL-UPS AS POSSIBLE (WITH OR WITHOUT A BAND, DEPENDING ON YOUR LEVEL)

WORKOUT 3 - SCALE OF POWER

3 X 5 OVERHEAD SQUATS (PAGE 100), 3 X 10 BARBELL AB ROLLOUTS (PAGE 190)

3 CLEANS (PAGE 34) AT 70 PERCENT OF MAXIMUM, 1 MINUTE OF REST, 3 MUSCLE-UPS (WITH OR WITHOUT A BAND, DEPENDING ON YOUR LEVEL), 1 MINUTE OF REST, 3 X 1 HEAVY SQUAT (PAGE 89) AND 1 JUMP WITHOUT THE BAR, 3 MINUTES OF REST

2 CLEANS AT 70 PERCENT OF MAXIMUM, 1 MINUTE OF REST, 2 MUSCLE-UPS (WITH OR WITHOUT A BAND, DEPENDING ON YOUR LEVEL), 1 MINUTE OF REST, 2 X 1 HEAVY SQUAT AND 1 JUMP WITHOUT THE BAR, 3 MINUTES OF REST

1 CLEAN AT 70 PERCENT OF MAXIMUM, 1 MINUTE OF REST, 1 MUSCLE-UP (WITH OR WITHOUT A BAND, DEPENDING ON YOUR LEVEL), 1 MINUTE OF REST, 1 X 1 HEAVY SQUAT AND 1 JUMP WITHOUT THE BAR, 3 MINUTES OF REST

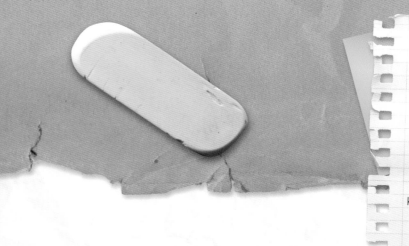

Technique tips

Begin while seated, crouching, or standing and try to reach as far as you can with the first hand. If possible, do this with a straight arm. Pull your body as high as possible (ideally, the hand should come almost all the way to the hip) before reaching with the other hand to repeat the move on the other side.

ROPE CLIMBING

Within the category of pulling exercises, rope climbing is the oldest exercise, yet it is also one of the most effective exercises, by a wide margin. Just like pull-ups, rope climbing heavily recruits all the muscles used in pulling, but it also provides additional benefits:

- Increased demand on the cardiovascular system
- A fun exercise
- Emphasis on training one side of the body at a time
- Movements at the shoulder occurring within a greater range of motion

The intense recruitment of the teres major, latissimus dorsi, biceps brachii, and the many forearm muscles—all of which are associated with performing any pulling movement—and the demanding load placed on the core musculature make this one of the most effective exercises for developing the upper limbs and torso.

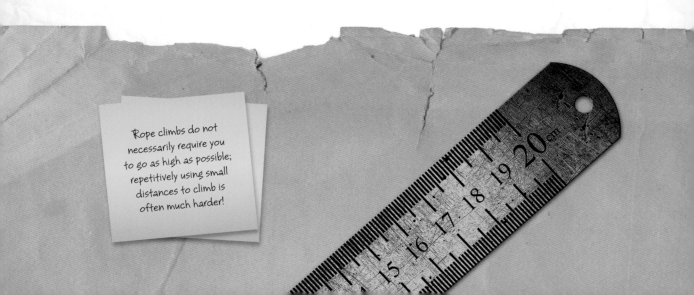

Rope climbs do not necessarily require you to go as high as possible; repetitively using small distances to climb is often much harder!

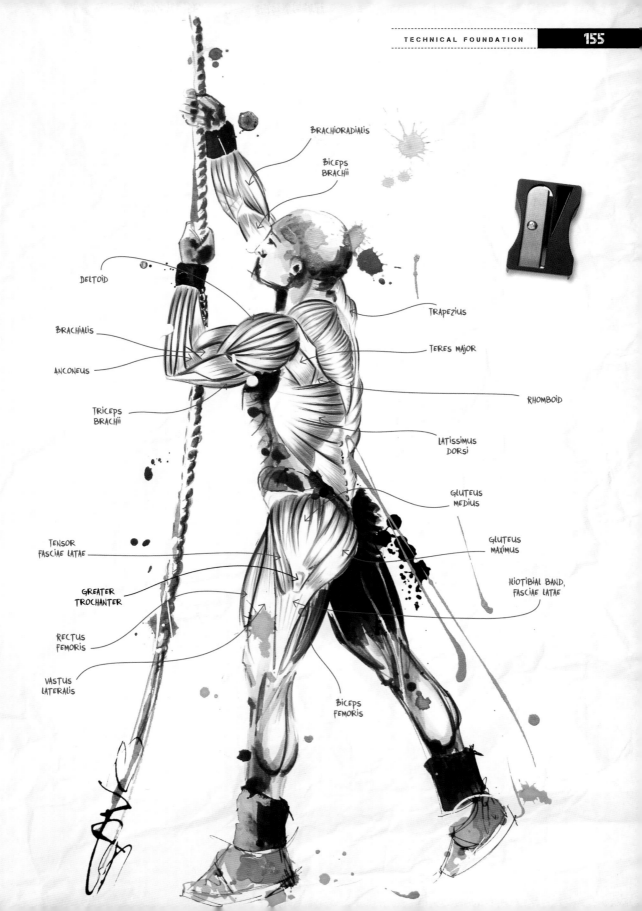

BRACHIORADIALIS

BICEPS BRACHII

DELTOID

BRACHIALIS

ANCONEUS

TRICEPS BRACHII

TENSOR FASCIAE LATAE

GREATER TROCHANTER

RECTUS FEMORIS

VASTUS LATERALIS

TRAPEZIUS

TERES MAJOR

RHOMBOID

LATISSIMUS DORSI

GLUTEUS MEDIUS

GLUTEUS MAXIMUS

ILIOTIBIAL BAND, FASCIAE LATAE

BICEPS FEMORIS

Beginning rope climbing

Starting to climb a rope can be difficult. Many beginners struggle mightily just to keep hanging on to the rope. If this is your case, you will have to adjust your training in the first few weeks until you can develop sufficient strength and proper technique. A good exercise to do first is working with the rope on the floor. Unroll the rope and lay it on a surface that is neither slippery nor sticky. Attach one end of the rope to a kettlebell or dumbbell and lie on your back at the other end of the rope. Then grab the rope and pull the weight toward your body. As you get stronger, increase the amount of weight. When you feel ready, try again to climb a vertical rope.

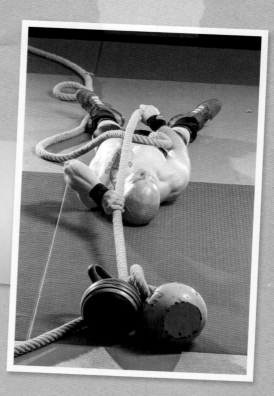

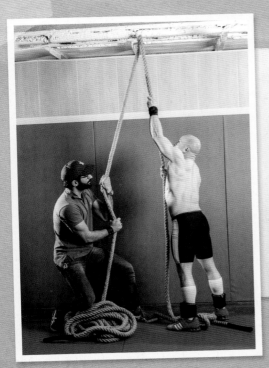

Another possibility is to develop strength specifically through eccentric exercises. By standing on a support or a bench close to the rope, you can train yourself to descend from the rope while controlling your speed. In this way, you remove the most difficult part of the exercise (the climb), but you are still practicing working with a rope. After a few sessions of eccentric work, you will be stronger and should be able to progress with the climbing portion of the exercise.

Finally, you can use a third method to help you overcome your body weight by keeping both feet firmly on the floor. This exercise is called the never-ending rope. You will need a partner. Pass the rope over a pull-up bar and ask your partner to hold onto one end. You pull on the other end as hard as you can, and your partner resists to slow down the sliding of the rope.

WORKOUT — ROPES

WORKOUT 1 — TIGHTROPE

AS FAST AS POSSIBLE: 5 ROUNDS OF 4 DEADLIFTS (PAGE 125), 2 ROPE CLIMBS, 20 SIT-UPS, 3 STRAIGHT-LEG DEADLIFTS (PAGE 136)

ADD-ON CIRCUIT FOR THE END OF THE WORKOUT, 3 ROUNDS: 4 SETS OF CORE EXERCISES, 40 SECONDS PER SET, 30 SECONDS OF RECOVERY BETWEEN SETS

WORKOUT 2 — TIGHTROPE WALKER

5 X 10 (MAX REPS) FRONT SQUATS (PAGE 97) AT 70 PERCENT OF MAXIMUM WITH NO MORE THAN 1 MINUTE OF REST

8 SETS OF ROPE CLIMBS: NORMAL ROPE CLIMB, 6 METERS WITH A 5-SECOND HOLD EVERY 2 METERS; NORMAL ROPE CLIMB, 6 METERS WHILE SLOWING YOUR DESCENT AS MUCH AS POSSIBLE; NORMAL ROPE CLIMB, 6 METERS EXPLOSIVELY (CLIMB AS FAST AS YOU CAN); NORMAL ROPE CLIMB, HANG FROM THE ROPE AS LONG AS YOU CAN.

4 X 10 REPS BARBELL AB ROLLOUTS (PAGE 190)

WORKOUT 3 — ROPE RUNNING

EVERY MINUTE FOR 12 MINUTES: 1 CLEAN AND JERK (PAGE 34), THEN, WITHOUT SETTING DOWN THE BAR, 2 FRONT SQUATS (PAGE 97), 5-METER ROPE CLIMB

THEN 5 X 5 BENCH PRESS (PAGE 121)

✖ PUSH-UP

The push-up has always been the first weapon in the fight to strengthen the upper body without equipment. This one exercise recruits the chest muscles, the triceps, and the anterior deltoid muscles.

Push-ups can be done from or to an inclined or declined surface (called incline or decline push-ups depending on the height of the hands or feet), which makes the exercise easier or harder and shifts the focus to certain aspects of the recruited muscles. The distance between the hands is important because it determines the load placed on the triceps (the closer the hands are to each other, the harder the triceps has to work). We recommend beginning with a hand placement that is most comfortable for you—in all likelihood, the one best suited for your body type.

You can also engage the triceps more if you rotate your hands slightly inward. The position of your feet is also something to consider, because when your feet are far apart, the exercise is easier.

If you are a beginner, do not hesitate to reduce the load by resting your knees on the ground.

You can also make the exercise harder by using a band wrapped snugly around your shoulders and under your hands.

Finally, stronger athletes can do push-ups supporting themselves on their fingers.

Technique tips

Position yourself facing the ground with your hands flat on the floor. You may place your hands however far apart is most comfortable for you. Be careful to keep your body in alignment. As much as possible, do not let your hips flex or your upper back round, because doing so can make your torso collapse inward. For proper form, contract your abdominal muscles and glutes tightly, stick out your chest, and keep your head in a neutral position. You must not arch your back or lower your head. Inhale and then lower your body as close to the floor as you can (so long as you have no shoulder discomfort). Exhale forcefully as you push yourself up.

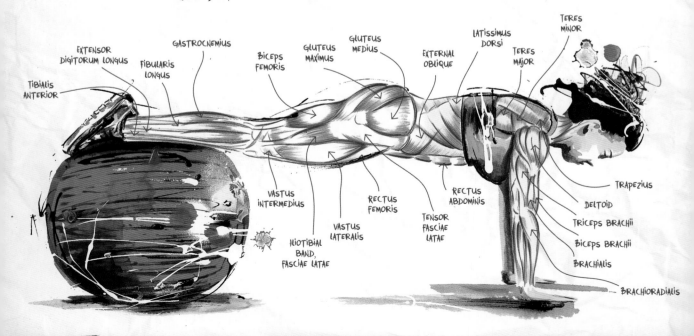

Normal push-ups

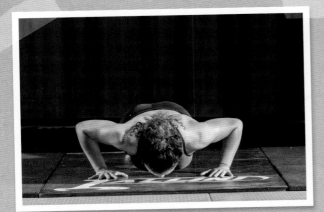
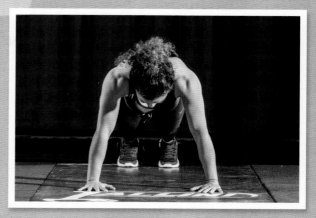

Decline push-ups

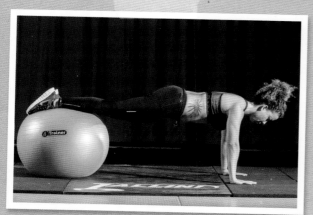
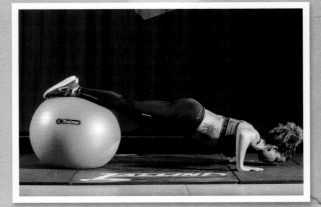

Incline push-ups

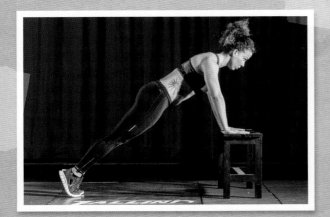
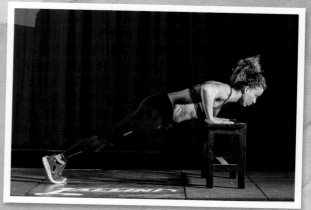

Push-ups on the fingers

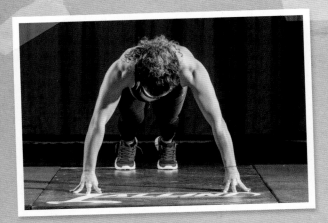

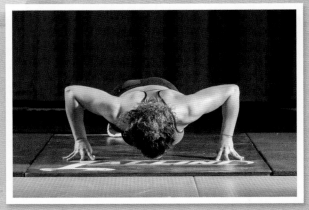

Narrow push-ups

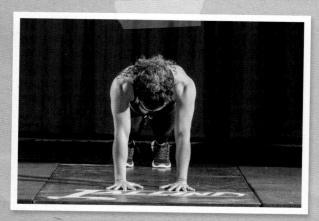

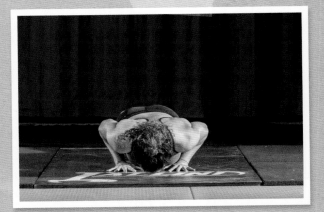

Wide push-ups

You can easily cheat when performing push-ups: Keep your body in alignment to optimize the effects of this exercise!

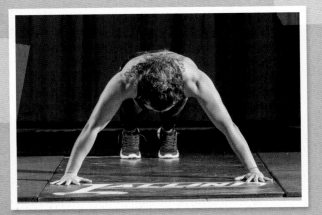

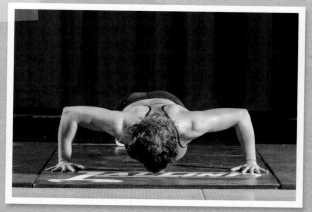

WORKOUT - PUSH-UPS

WORKOUT 1 - HOWLING PUSH-UPS

DO ONE SET OF PUSH-UPS UNTIL FAILURE. FOR SUBSEQUENT
SETS: SUBTRACT 2 PUSH-UPS FOR EACH SET UNTIL YOU REACH
20 AND THEN SUBTRACT 1 PUSH-UP FOR EVERY SET AFTER
THAT. TAKE ONLY 1 MINUTE OF REST MAXIMUM BETWEEN SETS.

FOR EXAMPLE, YOUR FIRST SET IS 24 PUSH-UPS, SO THE SECOND SET, 1
MINUTE LATER, IS 22 REPS, THE NEXT IS 20, THEN 19, 18, AND SO ON.

END WITH 10 X 10 ONE-LEGGED SQUATS (PAGE 108) AND 10 KNEE TUCK JUMPS.

WORKOUT 2 - PUSH, PUSH, PUSH

25 SQUATS (PAGE 89)
40 PUSH-UPS
20 SQUATS
32 PUSH-UPS
15 SQUATS
24 PUSH-UPS
10 SQUATS
16 PUSH-UPS
5 SQUATS
8 PUSH-UPS

WORKOUT 3 - 10 PUSH-UPS, 10 SECONDS

3 X 5 PISTOL SQUATS (PAGE 111) PER LEG

10 PUSH-UPS AND 10 SECONDS OF JUMPING IN PLACE OR JUMPING
ROPE; REPEAT UNTIL YOU ARE TOO TIRED TO CONTINUE

ADD-ON CIRCUIT: 6 MINUTES ALTERNATING 10 ABDOMINAL EXERCISES
AND 10 SIT-UPS NONSTOP, SWITCHING THE AB EXERCISE EACH TIME

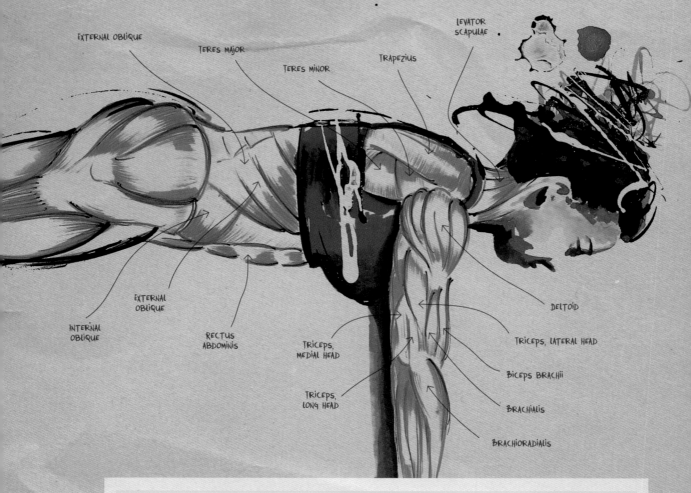

EXTERNAL OBLIQUE

TERES MAJOR

TERES MINOR

TRAPEZIUS

LEVATOR SCAPULAE

INTERNAL OBLIQUE

EXTERNAL OBLIQUE

RECTUS ABDOMINIS

TRICEPS, MEDIAL HEAD

TRICEPS, LONG HEAD

DELTOID

TRICEPS, LATERAL HEAD

BICEPS BRACHII

BRACHIALIS

BRACHIORADIALIS

RENEGADES

This set of exercises could also have been classified in the category of core exercises or pulling exercises.

The starting position is in a push-up with the hands holding on to two dumbbells or even two kettlebells. The three phases or positions of the exercise include the following:

- **Push-up**: Simply do a push-up while your hands are supported on parallel dumbbells.

- **Row**: Support yourself on one straight arm and bend the other elbow to bring the weight to your hip or your ribs.

- **Shoulder press**: Continue the pulling motion until your arm is stretched overhead. The top arm should be straight, and both arms should be in alignment. The head should remain in a neutral position.

For all of these, do not let the hips tilt forward or the upper back curve forward.

Keep your buttocks and abdominal muscles contracted throughout the exercise and open your chest to pull the shoulder blades together.

Finally, be sure to keep your body in alignment, especially by maintaining the hip extension. Feel free to combine the three movements within the same rep in any order you like.

①

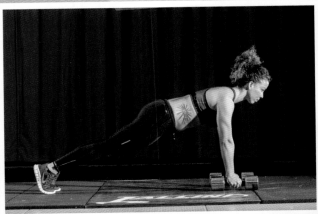

②

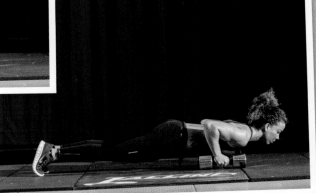

This exercise is shown here in its most complete form. You can also break it down into three phases or three exercise movements:
- Push-up
- Row
- Shoulder press

③

④

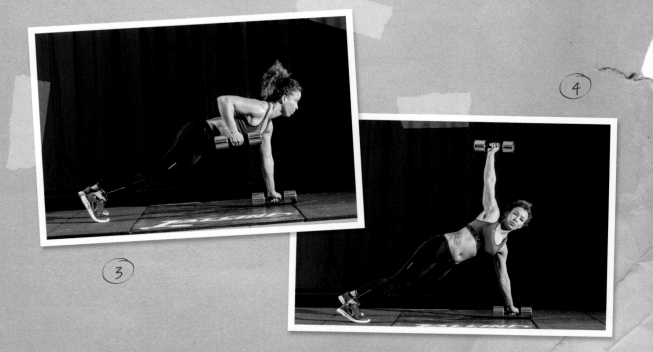

WORKOUT - RENEGADES

WORKOUT 1 - MEGAMIX

3 X 7 OVERHEAD SQUATS (PAGE 100), 3 X 5 FRONT SQUATS (PAGE 97)

10 SETS OF 10 RENEGADE PUSH-UPS, 10 RENEGADE ROWS,
10 SETS OF RENEGADE SHOULDER PRESSES

10 REPS OF THE COMPLETE RENEGADE (PUSH-UP,
ROW, AND SHOULDER PRESS)

WORKOUT 2 - RENEGADE JUSTICE

IN 20 MINUTES, DO AS MANY OF THE FOLLOWING CIRCUITS AS POSSIBLE:

10 PUSH-UPS AND RENEGADE ROWS, 10 THRUSTERS
(PAGE 103) WITH DUMBBELLS

WORKOUT 3 - RENEGADE FALL

21 RENEGADE ROWS, 21 DUMBBELL SQUATS

18 RENEGADE ROWS, 18 DUMBBELL SQUATS

15 RENEGADE ROWS, 15 DUMBBELL SQUATS

12 RENEGADE ROWS, 12 DUMBBELL SQUATS

9 RENEGADE ROWS, 9 DUMBBELL SQUATS

5 RENEGADE ROWS, 5 DUMBBELL SQUATS

3 RENEGADE ROWS, 3 DUMBBELL SQUATS

1 RENEGADE ROW, 1 DUMBBELL SQUAT

BURPEE

This dynamic exercise combines a squat, push-up, and a jump that are performed in quick succession. The exercise can be divided into parts with three levels of difficulty:

➲ **With straight arms (like a plank)**: focuses on shoulder stability and helps increase speed when the primary focus of the workout is metabolic endurance, not muscular endurance

➲ **With a push-up**: adds greater stress on the upper-body muscles than just holding the plank position

➲ **With a jump (a knee tuck or an X-jump)**: a complete version that requires the lower body to generate power for the jump, thereby applying muscular and metabolic demands on the whole body

For a complete burpee, from a standing position, squat down rapidly, kick your legs backward to get into a plank position, perform a push-up, tuck your legs back under your body, and jump back up to a standing position as quickly as possible.

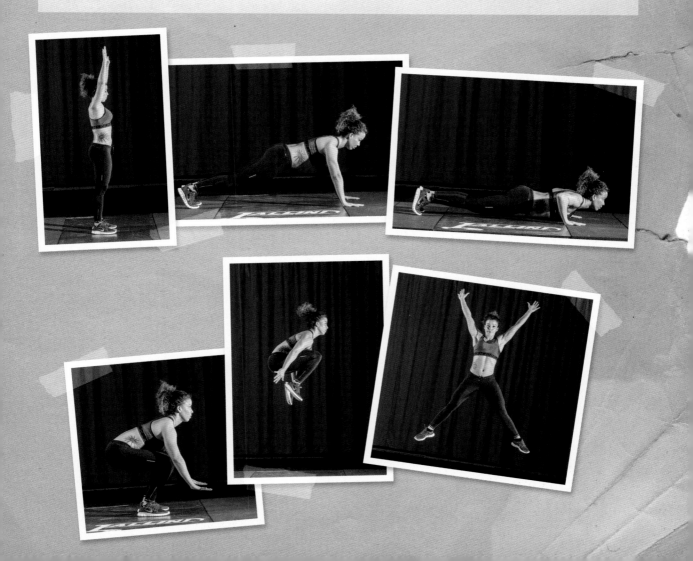

WORKOUT - BURPEES

WORKOUT 1 - THE PLAGUES OF EGYPT

AS FAST AS POSSIBLE:

400-METER SPRINT

50 JUMPING LUNGES

40 PLANK BURPEES

30 ITWS (PAGE 30)

20 PUSH-UP BURPEES AND PULL-UPS (PAGE 143)

10 OVERHEAD SQUATS (PAGE 100)

20 COMPLETE BURPEES AND PULL-UPS

30 ITWS

WORKOUT 2 - DOUBLE CHEESE

REPEAT THIS COMBINATION 100 TIMES AS FAST AS YOU CAN:
2 PUSH-UPS (PAGE 158), 2 COMPLETE BURPEES, 2 PULL-UPS (PAGE 143)

WORKOUT 3 - TABLE FOR 12

12 ROUNDS:

12 PUSH-UPS (PAGE 158)

12 COMPLETE BURPEES

12 PULL-UPS (PAGE 143)

CLAPPING PUSH-UP

In this explosive push-up, you must quickly push off from the floor high enough so that you can clap your hands. The same variations used with regular push-ups work here too. You can also change the height of your hands or only one hand if you use steps or a medicine ball.

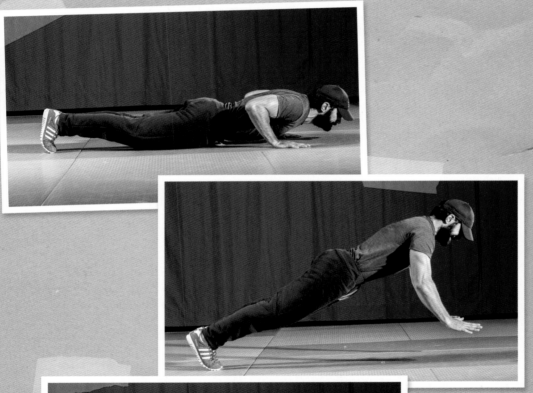

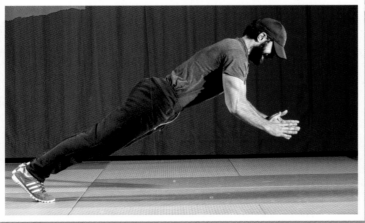

Push-ups are as much a strengthening exercise for the upper body as they are a core exercise; strive to keep your body in alignment.

WORKOUT – CLAPPING PUSH-UPS

WORKOUT 1 – THE LESS YOU SQUAT, THE MORE YOU PUSH

5 X 3 DEADLIFTS (PAGE 125) COMBINED WITH 6 CLAPPING PULL-UPS (PAGE 148), RECOVERY: 2 MINUTES

10 SQUATS (PAGE 89), 5 CLAPPING PUSH-UPS, 15 DEADLIFTS

8 SQUATS, 7 CLAPPING PUSH-UPS, 12 DEADLIFTS

6 SQUATS, 9 CLAPPING PUSH-UPS, 9 DEADLIFTS

4 SQUATS, 11 CLAPPING PUSH-UPS, 6 DEADLIFTS

2 SQUATS, AS MANY CLAPPING PUSH-UPS AS POSSIBLE, 4 DEADLIFTS

WORKOUT 2 – FINAL CLAP

4 X 8 SQUATS (PAGE 89) AT YOUR 8-REP MAX WITH 90 SECONDS OF REST

4 X 8 WEIGHTED PULL-UPS (PAGE 143) AT YOUR 8-REP MAX WITH 90 SECONDS OF REST

4 ROUNDS AS FAST AS POSSIBLE: 15 CLAPPING PUSH-UPS, 30 KNEE TUCK JUMPS

WORKOUT 3 – STARTING CLAP

5 FRONT SQUATS (PAGE 97), 3 MINUTES OF REST, 5 SQUATS (PAGE 89), 3 MINUTES OF REST, 5 FRONT SQUATS (PAGE 97), 3 MINUTES OF REST, 5 SQUATS, 3 MINUTES OF REST

7 SETS OF 8 ALTERNATING CLAPPING PUSH-UPS (USING A STEP), STRIVING TO REACH YOUR MAXIMUM HEIGHT, THEN A 50-METER SPRINT, RECOVERY: 4 MINUTES

✖ EXPLOSIVE PUSH-UP
DOUBLE KNEE TUCK PUSH-UP

This is the hardest version of clapping push-ups. This time, you push off the ground and bring your legs and arms together before returning to the starting position. An even harder version involves doing a half turn during the knee tuck. This exercise combines extra abdominal work with with the intensity of an explosive push-up.

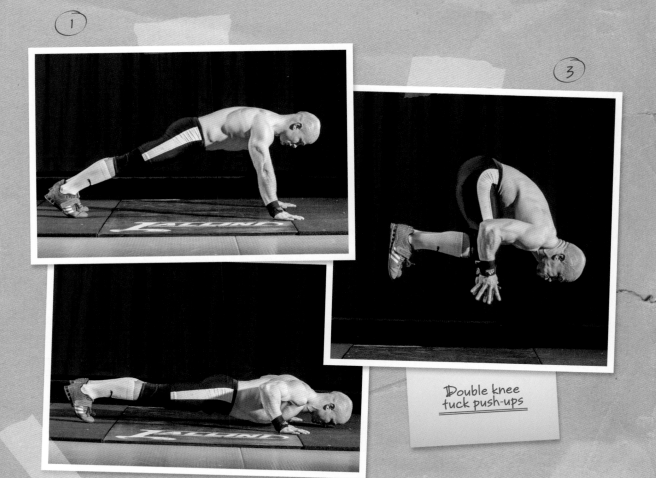

Double knee tuck push-ups

Key points for the double knee tuck push-up:

1. Strive for maximum acceleration as your arms extend.
2. Tuck the knees as high and as quickly as possible.
3. Control your body alignment as you land.

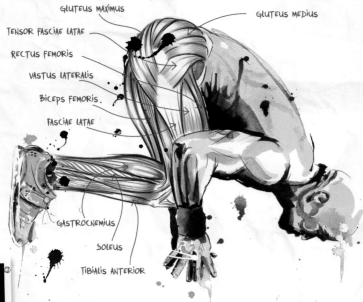

Note that the psoas inserts on the lumbar spine (see the following page). Therefore, body alignment could be compromised during certain wide-open exercises. Watch the placement of your back and pelvis in exercises in which your torso and legs are far apart.

GLUTEUS MAXIMUS
GLUTEUS MEDIUS
TENSOR FASCIAE LATAE
RECTUS FEMORIS
VASTUS LATERALIS
BICEPS FEMORIS
FASCIAE LATAE
GASTROCNEMIUS
SOLEUS
TIBIALIS ANTERIOR

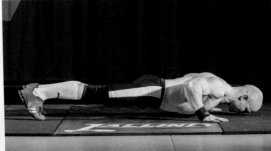

1

Half-rotation push-ups

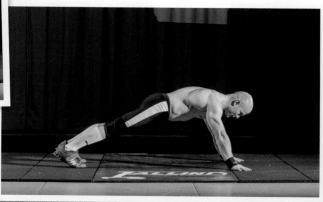

2

3

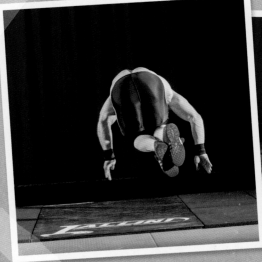

4

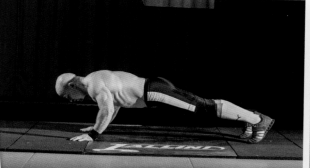

Here the pushing speed must be even faster than in double knee tuck push-ups; try to go as fast and as high as possible.

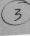

AZTEC PUSH-UP

Just as in double knee tuck push-ups, the trick here is to generate enough power to bring the straight legs and torso together in the air. Bringing the torso and legs together recruits the abdominal muscles, hip flexors, and erector spinae even more. The large amount of force that must be generated, combined with dynamic stability work in all the regions of the spine in a short amount of time, results in an incredible amount of muscle recruitment for an exercise that does not require any additional weight.

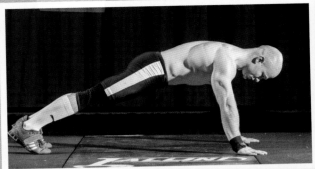

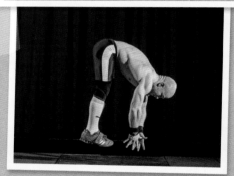

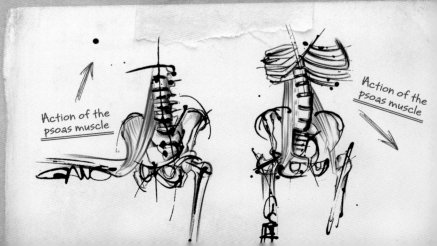

The psoas is strengthened as much as it is stretched. Take the time to stretch your psoas before exposing it to this kind of tension.

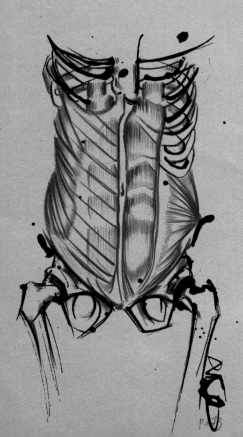

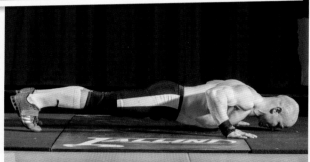

Action of the psoas muscle

Action of the psoas muscle

SUPERMAN PUSH-UP

Following the same principles as the double knee tuck push-up and the Aztec push-up, this time the force generated should allow you to hold your body horizontally (parallel to the floor). Again, muscle recruitment alternates between maximum power and stability.

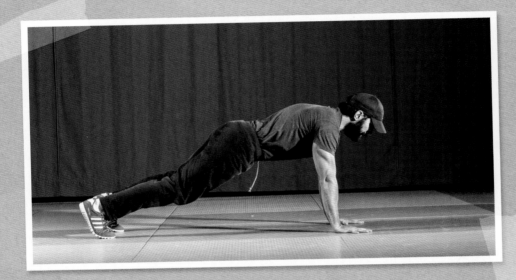

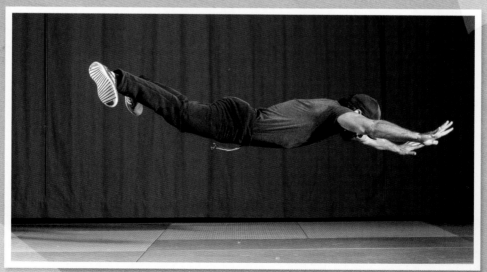

This advanced exercise is not for beginners.

WORKOUT – EXPLOSIVE PUSH-UPS

WORKOUT 1 – SHADOKS

10 MINUTES, STARTING EVERY MINUTE:
5 KETTLEBELL SNATCHES PER ARM (PAGE 76)
5 COMPLETE BURPEES (PAGE 165)
RECOVERY: 4 MINUTES

THEN FOR 10 MINUTES,
STARTING EVERY MINUTE:
5 TWO-HANDED KETTLEBELL
SWINGS (HEAVY, PAGE 128)
4 DOUBLE KNEE TUCK PUSH-UPS WITH A
HALF AND THEN A QUARTER ROTATION

WORKOUT 2 – PUSH-UP STRIKE

4 ROUNDS: 10 SQUATS (PAGE 89), 15
SECONDS OF JUMPING ROPE, 10 KNEE TUCK
JUMPS, 15 SECONDS OF JUMPING ROPE

BEGIN WITH AN EXPLOSIVE DOUBLE KNEE
TUCK PUSH-UP WITH A HALF ROTATION.
THEN ADD 1 PUSH-UP EVERY 30 SECONDS,
FIRST WITH A HALF ROTATION. THEN, AS YOU
GET TIRED, SWITCH TO REGULAR DOUBLE
KNEE TUCK PUSH-UPS, THEN CLAPPING
PUSH-UPS, AND THEN REGULAR PUSH-
UPS. CONTINUE UNTIL YOU REACH FAILURE.

WORKOUT 3 – FEELING GOOD ABOUT PUSH-UPS

100-METER RUN
15 PUSH-UPS (PAGE 158)
5 COMPLETE BURPEES (PAGE 165)
2 PUSH-UPS WITH A HALF ROTATION
100-METER RUN
10 PUSH-UPS
5 COMPLETE BURPEES
10 CLAPPING PUSH-UPS
5 PUSH-UP BURPEES
100-METER RUN
20 PUSH-UPS
5 COMPLETE BURPEES
5 DOUBLE KNEE TUCK OR
AZTEC PUSH-UPS
5 PUSH-UP BURPEES
100-METER RUN
8 PUSH-UPS
5 PUSH-UP BURPEES
5 SUPERMAN PUSH-UPS
5 COMPLETE BURPEES
10 PUSH-UPS ON THE FINGERS
100-METER RUN

✖ BATTLE ROPES

Battle ropes can also be used horizontally to develop metabolic endurance and strength. You can shift the focus of the exercise by using ropes with different lengths, weights, and thicknesses. Technique tips: bent legs, back straight, torso leaning forward, head up, and gaze fixed on a point at the horizon. Other versions: waves with one or two hands; small, medium, or large waves; side waves; crossed ropes or underhand grip; and raised to the side (star). You can add leg work later as your coordination improves.

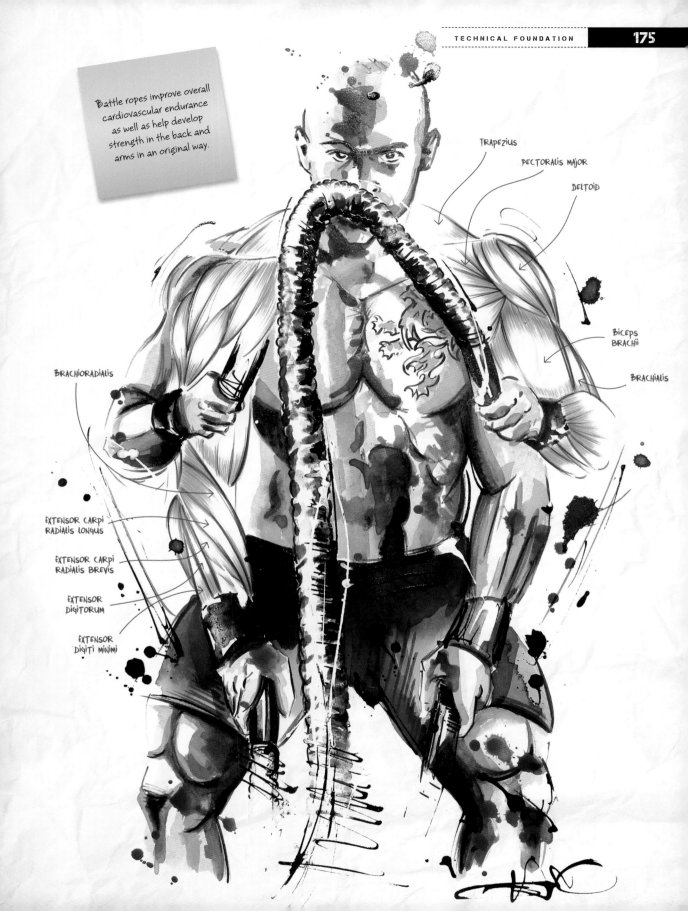

Battle ropes improve overall cardiovascular endurance as well as help develop strength in the back and arms in an original way.

TRAPEZIUS

PECTORALIS MAJOR

DELTOID

BICEPS BRACHII

BRACHIALIS

BRACHIORADIALIS

EXTENSOR CARPI RADIALIS LONGUS

EXTENSOR CARPI RADIALIS BREVIS

EXTENSOR DIGITORUM

EXTENSOR DIGITI MINIMI

Keep the legs
slightly bent.

Normal waves
at different
heights

All these
exercises can
be modified
by moving the
feet from the
front to the
back, to the
side, or into a
lunge position.

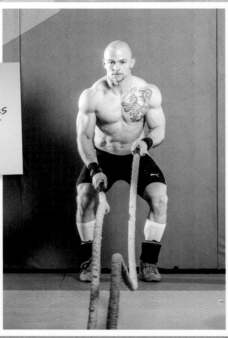

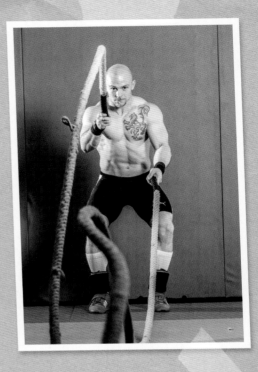

Keep firm
control over
the position
of your back
even though it
is not directly
supporting
any weight.

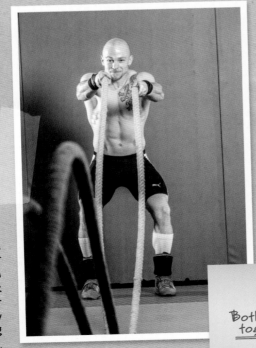

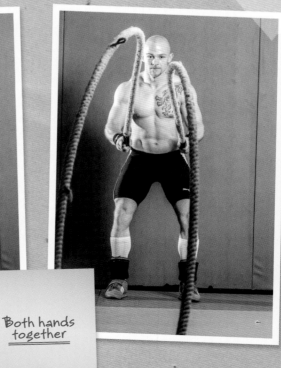

Both hands
together

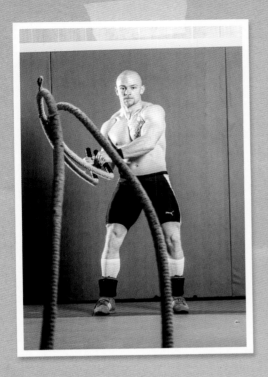

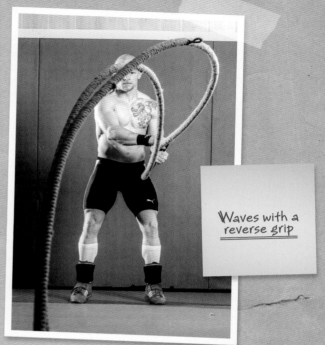

Waves with a reverse grip

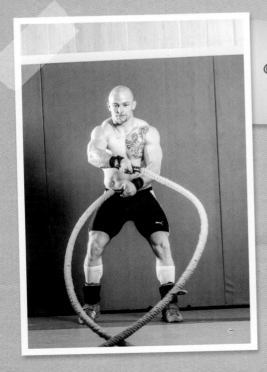

Crossing waves

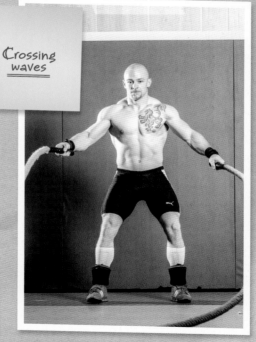

Feel free to vary all these exercises in your workout.

①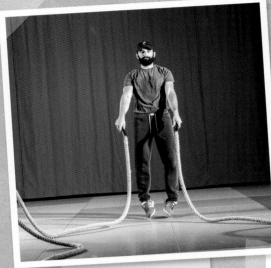

②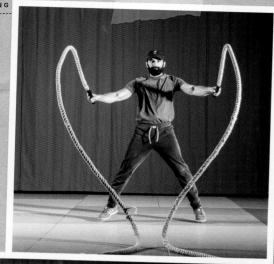

Star
waves

③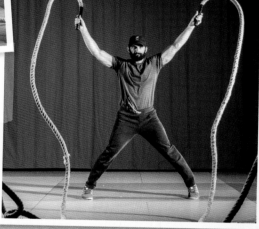

Table summarizing
the various effects of
battle rope exercises.

	Cardio	Strength	Coordination	Core
Normal wave	**	**	*	*
Small wave	***	*	**	*
Large wave	**	**	**	**
Both hands together	*	***	*	**
Reverse grip	*	**	**	***
Crossing waves	*	*	***	**
Star waves	**	*	***	*

WORKOUT - BATTLE ROPES

WORKOUT 1 - RUSSIAN MOUNTAINS

3 X 10 BOX JUMPS, 3 X 10 KNEE TUCK JUMPS,
3 X 10 COMPLETE BURPEES (PAGE 165)

DO FOR 10 MINUTES: 20 SECONDS OF NORMAL BATTLE ROPE
WAVES, 20-METER SPRINT (RUN, COME BACK 2 X 10 METERS),
10 COMPLETE BURPEES, 20 SECONDS OF BATTLE ROPE WAVES
WITH BOTH HANDS, 10 KNEE TUCK JUMPS, 10 X-JUMP BURPEES

10 X 30 SECONDS FAST RUN, 30 SECONDS SLOW RUN

WORKOUT 2 - MULTIPLE ENDS

DO 6 ROUNDS AS FAST AS POSSIBLE: 10 KNEE TUCK JUMPS,
10 BATTLE ROPE WAVES WITH BOTH HANDS, 10 PLANK BURPEES
(PAGE 165), 10 BATTLE ROPE LARGE WAVES, 400-METER RUN

WORKOUT 3 - SONIC WAVE

EVERY MINUTE FOR 10 MINUTES: WAVE THE BATTLE
ROPES AS FAST AS POSSIBLE FOR 10 SECONDS

10 ROUNDS: 10 BATTLE ROPE WAVES WITH BOTH
HANDS, 5 PUSH-UP BURPEES (PAGE 165), 50-METER
SPRINT AT MAX SPEED, RECOVERY: 3 MINUTES

✖ DIPS

Another classic exercise, dips on parallel bars, heavily recruits the pectoral, triceps, and deltoids muscles. The simplicity of dips means they are a logical choice for high intensity training circuits, but that does not mean they are less technical. They often end up being done with poor form. The athlete who uses poor form risks the kinds of shoulder injuries described elsewhere in this book.

Dips are also sometimes done using rings, which increase muscle recruitment (such as by including the latissimus dorsi) because of the inherent instability of the rings.

DELTOID

TRICEPS BRACHII

SERRATUS ANTERIOR

PECTORALIS MAJOR

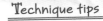

Technique tips

Your arms should be straight, your hands should be on the bars, and your shoulders should be just in front of your hands. Keep your head in a neutral and comfortable position (do not look at the ground and round your back and do not lift your head too high). Bend your arms to lower your body, but keep your body as vertical as you can (avoid any swinging or diagonal positions). When your shoulders are at the level of the elbows, come back up by pushing against the bars but keep your trajectory as vertical as possible.

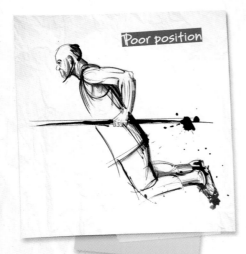

Poor position

WORKOUT - Dips

WORKOUT 1 - Dip the Box

21, 15, 9 reps of deadlifts (page 125), box jumps, dips

Then as many pull-ups (page 143) as possible in 5 minutes

Then as many squats (page 89) at 40
percent as possible in 5 minutes

WORKOUT 2 - Dip Squat

4 x 6 squats (page 89)

Every minute for 15 minutes: 3 cleans (page 34), 8 dips

WORKOUT 3 - Weight Dipping

10 x 1 snatches (page 60) every minute

Bent-over rows (page 83) 3 x 5

As many times as possible in 8 minutes:
6 dips, 10 kettlebell swings (page 128)

✖ CORE EXERCISES

Besides squats and weightlifting movements that require a certain level of functional core stability, many exercises dedicated to core stability are now part of high intensity training. The list of potential exercises coming from gymnastics, bodybuilding, and conditioning is almost infinite. Here we include only the classics.

When the gap between the torso and the legs is too large, it can interfere with body alignment and put the lumbar region at risk.

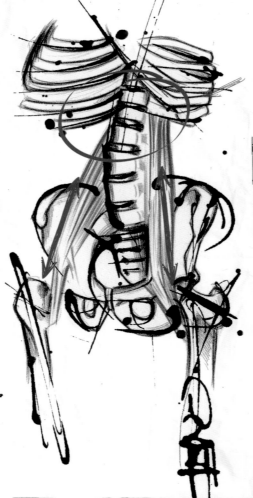

The psoas muscles insert at the lumbar spine and dig into the lumbar curve when they are lengthened or shortened.

V-UP

This version of a sit-up probably provides the most intense rectus abdominis recruitment of any exercise available. The distance between the distal loads (here, the arms and the legs) has a maximum effect and generates an unusual level of abdominal muscle tension. The iliopsoas muscles and hip flexors are also heavily recruited.

Position of the hip
in the different
stages of a V-up

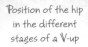

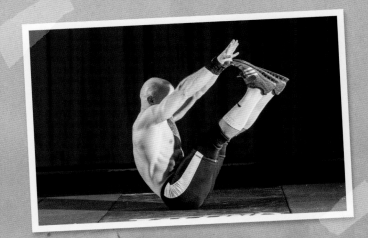

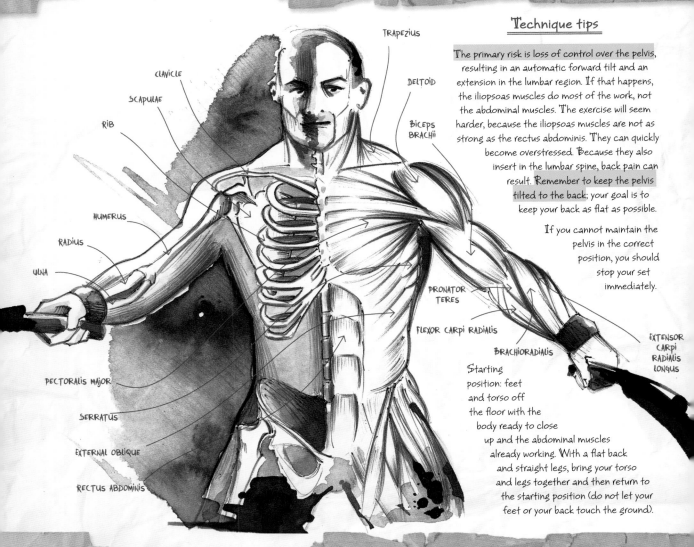

Technique tips

The primary risk is loss of control over the pelvis, resulting in an automatic forward tilt and an extension in the lumbar region. If that happens, the iliopsoas muscles do most of the work, not the abdominal muscles. The exercise will seem harder, because the iliopsoas muscles are not as strong as the rectus abdominis. They can quickly become overstressed. Because they also insert in the lumbar spine, back pain can result. Remember to keep the pelvis tilted to the back; your goal is to keep your back as flat as possible.

If you cannot maintain the pelvis in the correct position, you should stop your set immediately.

TRAPEZIUS

CLAVICLE

SCAPULAE

RIB

DELTOID

BICEPS BRACHII

HUMERUS

RADIUS

ULNA

PRONATOR TERES

FLEXOR CARPI RADIALIS

BRACHIORADIALIS

EXTENSOR CARPI RADIALIS LONGUS

PECTORALIS MAJOR

SERRATUS

EXTERNAL OBLIQUE

RECTUS ABDOMINIS

Starting position: feet and torso off the floor with the body ready to close up and the abdominal muscles already working. With a flat back and straight legs, bring your torso and legs together and then return to the starting position (do not let your feet or your back touch the ground).

WORKOUT - V-UPS

WORKOUT 1 - VITALLI

5 X 20 METERS OF FORWARD LUNGES (PAGE 140), 20 METERS
OF BACKWARD LUNGES, RECOVERY: MAX 2 MINUTES

AS MANY REPS AS POSSIBLE AT 65 PERCENT OF YOUR MAX IN THE
SQUAT (PAGE 89), BENCH PRESS (PAGE 121), AND DEADLIFT (PAGE 125)
(1 SET OF EACH WITH 2 MINUTES OF RECOVERY BETWEEN SETS)

THEN 3 ROUNDS OF 400 METERS AND AS MANY
V-UPS AS POSSIBLE, RECOVERY: 3 MINUTES

WORKOUT 2 - ISAAC

4 ROUNDS:

AS MANY DEADLIFTS (PAGE 125) AS POSSIBLE
IN 1 MINUTE, RECOVERY: 1 MINUTE

AS MANY V-UPS AS POSSIBLE IN 1 MINUTE, RECOVERY: 1 MINUTE

AS MANY PULL-UPS (PAGE 143) AS POSSIBLE IN 1 MINUTE, RECOVERY: 1 MINUTE

FINISH WITH 100 PUSH-UPS (PAGE 158) IN THE
SMALLEST NUMBER OF SETS POSSIBLE

WORKOUT 3 - ABS AND RACES

3 ROUNDS IN AS LITTLE TIME AS POSSIBLE:

600-METER RUN, 20 TOES TO BAR (PAGE
185), 300-METER RUN, 20 V-UPS

TOES TO BAR

Toes to bar is another popular exercise used in high intensity training programs. This vertical variation of a V-up stresses the arm and back muscles and heavily works the rectus abdominis and iliopsoas muscles.

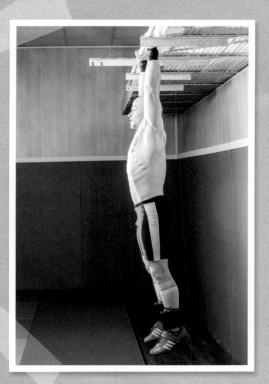 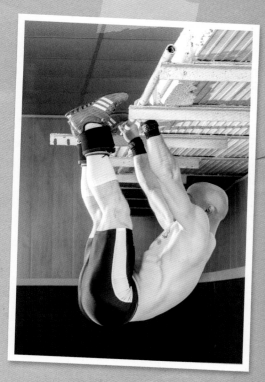

Technique tips

Hang from the bar with straight arms, raise your toes to the bar while keeping your legs straight, and then lower the legs back down. Absolutely no swinging or momentum should be present. You must lower your legs with control. The eccentric phase, as the pelvis is opened, should be done with control, not only to make the exercise more effective, but also for your safety. The pelvis should never swing forward.

WORKOUT – TOES TO BAR

WORKOUT 1 – CLIFFHANGER

1 SQUAT (PAGE 89) AND 1 DEADLIFT (PAGE 125), RECOVERY: 1 MINUTE
2 SQUATS AND 2 DEADLIFTS, RECOVERY: 90 SECONDS
3 SQUATS AND 3 DEADLIFTS, RECOVERY: 2 MINUTES
THEN, EVERY MINUTE FOR 10 MINUTES:
3 X 1 PULL-UP (PAGE 143) AND 5 TOES TO BAR

WORKOUT 2 – DWIGHT

DO THE FOLLOWING CIRCUIT 3 TIMES:
1 MINUTE OF PUSH-UPS (PAGE 158)
1 MINUTE OF A SNATCH (PAGE 60) AND 2 KNEE TUCK JUMPS
1 MINUTE OF COMPLETE BURPEES (PAGE 165)
1 MINUTE OF TOES TO BAR
1 MINUTE ELBOW PLANK
1 MINUTE OF PULL-UPS (PAGE 143)
2 MINUTES OF RECOVERY BETWEEN CIRCUITS

WORKOUT 3 – JOSHUA

4 ROUNDS
AS MANY DEADLIFTS (PAGE 125) AS POSSIBLE
IN 1 MINUTE, RECOVERY: 1 MINUTE
AS MANY TOES TO BAR AS POSSIBLE IN 1 MINUTE, RECOVERY: 1 MINUTE
AS MANY PUSH-UPS (PAGE 158) AS POSSIBLE
IN 1 MINUTE, RECOVERY: 1 MINUTE
TO FINISH, 100 PULL-UPS (PAGE 143) IN A MINIMUM NUMBER OF SETS

TURKISH GET-UP

This exercise is one of the most complete dynamic exercises for the body. It combines intense abdominal strengthening with shoulder stability, strengthening of the lower limbs, and isometric arm work.

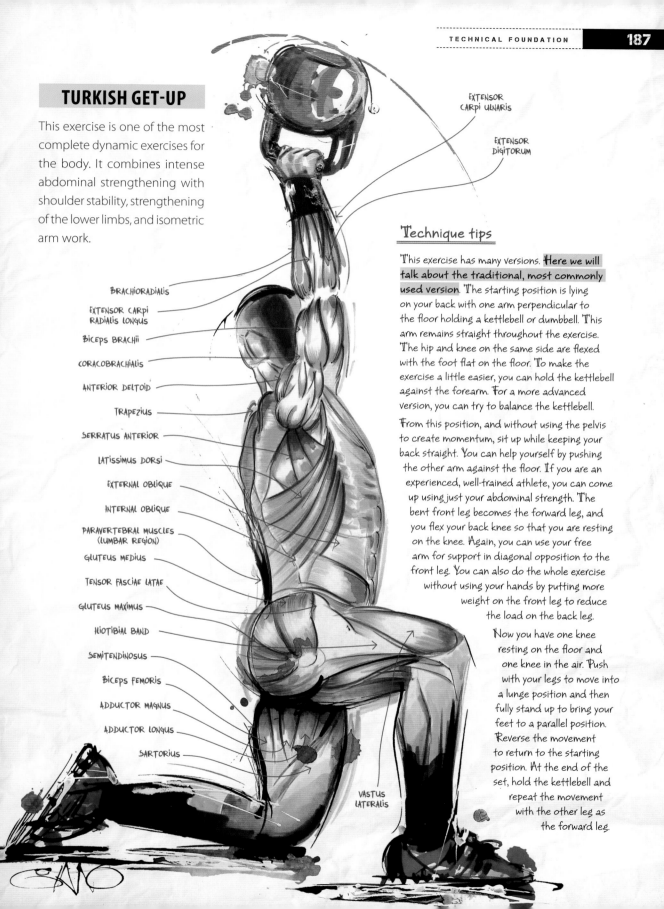

EXTENSOR CARPI ULNARIS

EXTENSOR DIGITORUM

BRACHIORADIALIS

EXTENSOR CARPI RADIALIS LONGUS

BICEPS BRACHII

CORACOBRACHIALIS

ANTERIOR DELTOID

TRAPEZIUS

SERRATUS ANTERIOR

LATISSIMUS DORSI

EXTERNAL OBLIQUE

INTERNAL OBLIQUE

PARAVERTEBRAL MUSCLES (LUMBAR REGION)

GLUTEUS MEDIUS

TENSOR FASCIAE LATAE

GLUTEUS MAXIMUS

ILIOTIBIAL BAND

SEMITENDINOSUS

BICEPS FEMORIS

ADDUCTOR MAGNUS

ADDUCTOR LONGUS

SARTORIUS

VASTUS LATERALIS

Technique tips

This exercise has many versions. Here we will talk about the traditional, most commonly used version. The starting position is lying on your back with one arm perpendicular to the floor holding a kettlebell or dumbbell. This arm remains straight throughout the exercise. The hip and knee on the same side are flexed with the foot flat on the floor. To make the exercise a little easier, you can hold the kettlebell against the forearm. For a more advanced version, you can try to balance the kettlebell.

From this position, and without using the pelvis to create momentum, sit up while keeping your back straight. You can help yourself by pushing the other arm against the floor. If you are an experienced, well-trained athlete, you can come up using just your abdominal strength. The bent front leg becomes the forward leg, and you flex your back knee so that you are resting on the knee. Again, you can use your free arm for support in diagonal opposition to the front leg. You can also do the whole exercise without using your hands by putting more weight on the front leg to reduce the load on the back leg.

Now you have one knee resting on the floor and one knee in the air. Push with your legs to move into a lunge position and then fully stand up to bring your feet to a parallel position. Reverse the movement to return to the starting position. At the end of the set, hold the kettlebell and repeat the movement with the other leg as the forward leg.

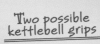

Two possible
kettlebell grips

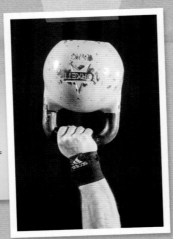

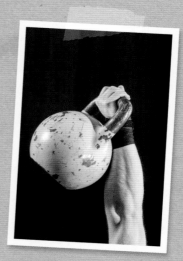

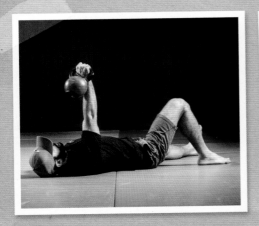

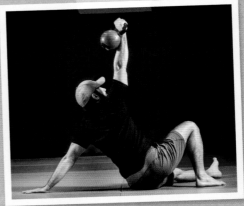

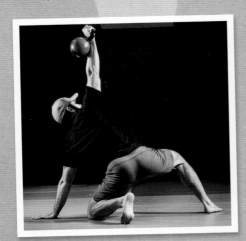

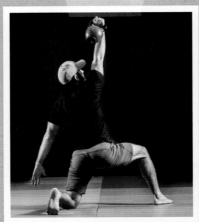

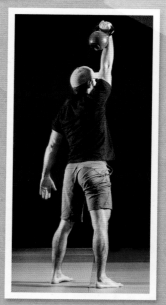

WORKOUT – TURKISH GET-UPS

WORKOUT 1 – READY FOR TERRITORY ACTION

DO THE FOLLOWING CIRCUIT 3 TIMES:

1 MINUTE OF DIPS (PAGE 180)

1 MINUTE OF CLEAN (PAGE 34) AND OVER THE BAR JUMP, HALF ROTATION

1 MINUTE OF BURPEES (PAGE 165)

1 MINUTE OF TURKISH GET-UPS, SWITCHING HANDS

1-MINUTE ROPE CLIMB (PAGE 154) TO 3 METERS (TOUCH THE FEET ON THE FLOOR AFTER EACH REP)

1-MINUTE ELBOW PLANK

2 MINUTES OF RECOVERY BETWEEN CIRCUITS

WORKOUT 2 – I AIN'T MAD AT 'CHA

5 ROUNDS:

400-METER RUN, 1 ROPE CLIMB TO 4 METERS (PAGE 154), 10 TURKISH GET-UPS (5 ON THE RIGHT AND 5 ON THE LEFT), 10 V-UPS (PAGE 184)

WORKOUT 3 – THE WRATH OF THE TITANS

5 ROPE CLIMBS (PAGE 154) TO 3 METERS

THEN AS MANY TIMES AS POSSIBLE IN 20 MINUTES:
8 TURKISH GET-UPS ALTERNATING RIGHT AND LEFT ARMS, 5 PULL-UPS (WITH BAND ASSIST, PAGE 143), 10 COMPLETE BURPEES (PAGE 165)

BARBELL AB ROLLOUT

Barbell ab rollouts are an intense exercise that works the entire core from the shoulders to the pelvis including the entire spine.

Advanced version

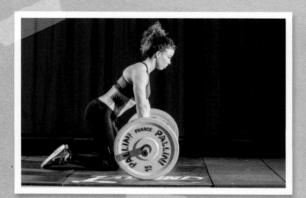

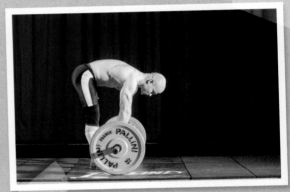

Be sure not to round your back

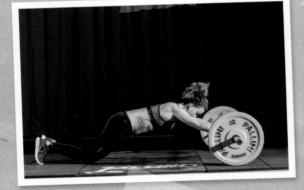

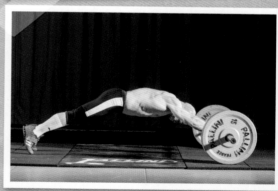

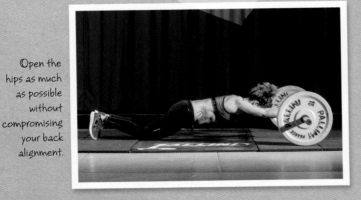

Open the hips as much as possible without compromising your back alignment.

Technique tips

Begin in a push-up position with a bar with a rotating sleeve and loaded with weight plates on the floor. You can rest your knees on the floor or hold them in the air to make the exercise harder. Roll the bar forward, keeping all the parts of your body in proper alignment. You should have a nearly complete hip extension, and if the knees are in the air, they must be fully extended as well. Squeeze the shoulder blades together without arching the back. Push out the chest slightly and keep the head in line with the spine. Lower as far as you can (if possible, with arms fully extended). Follow these same principles and return to the starting position.

WORKOUT – BARBELL AB ROLLOUTS

WORKOUT 1 – ROLLERCOASTER

5 ROUNDS:

8 DEADLIFTS AT 50 PERCENT OF MAXIMUM (PAGE 125), 50-METER RUN, 8 BARBELL AB ROLLOUTS, 50-METER RUN, 10 KNEE TUCK JUMPS, 50-METER RUN

WORKOUT 2 – RANGUIROA

10 ROUNDS:

5 SQUATS (PAGE 89) AT 70 PERCENT OF MAXIMUM

5 BARBELL AB ROLLOUTS

10 KNEE TUCK JUMPS

10 V-UPS (PAGE 184)

WORKOUT 3 – SIN CITY

EVERY MINUTE FOR 10 MINUTES: 1 CLEAN (PAGE 34), 1 BENCH PRESS (PAGE 121), 1 BARBELL AB ROLLOUT

THEN 5 ROUNDS OF 5 LIGHT CLEANS (PAGE 34), 7 DEADLIFTS (PAGE 125), 4 DOUBLE KNEE TUCK JUMPS AND PUSH-UPS (PAGE 158)

RUNNING

No high intensity training program would be complete without a running component. Incorporating running into your warm-up not only improves performance and reduces injuries but also helps you to . . . run faster!

Here you will find a more detailed explanation of running technique as well as drills that can help you improve your technique. As always, at the end of the chapter, you can get inspiration by exploring specific running workouts for your daily training.

RUNNING TECHNIQUES

Using the term fundamental to refer to normal skills is somewhat of a paradox. In fact, we could consider athletic drills as fundamental to running and running as one of the fundamentals of more advanced types of training.

The catch is that running is, at least in appearance, the most easily accessible type of training. Indeed, you do not have to learn how to run to compete against others in the schoolyard. In any case, when a beginner starts to do high intensity training workouts, he or she will probably be more focused on mastering snatches from a weightlifting rack. But something changes the moment we move beyond the fun aspect of so-called functional running and devote ourselves to a training activity motivated by performance and progress. We move from running just to move quickly to a style of running that is a true technical practice enhanced by biomechanical and bioenergetic input. Learning this requires specific training methods.

Just as in weightlifting, the beginner methods will become, once automated, an expert's specific warm-up drills. Do not get ahead of yourself; if you are a beginner, take the time to learn and master these drills so that they can later become an integral part of your workout.

Only after you have internalized all the finer points will you be able to use these drills as warm-up routines. The fundamentals are the basics that a runner must master, no matter the distance to be run (the drills can later be slightly modified or supplemented depending on the distance and the speed as well as the running conditions: track or street running, cushioned or minimalist shoes, and so on):

- **Torso upright**: Remove any trace of rounded or hyperextended posture.

- **Contralateral synchronization of arms and legs**: As the left leg moves forward, the right arm is activated in a synchronous movement and vice versa.

- **Control the pelvis**: The pelvis should be supported and tilted slightly to the back. Avoid any exaggeration of the lumbar curve.

- **Support your weight on the front of the foot**: Avoid braking into the running surface with your heel each time you land.

The role of the hips is essential, so the psoas muscle is at the heart of your balance and helps drive the movement. Respecting these basic truths is important both from a conditioning point of view and for performance.

A TOTAL-BODY APPROACH TO RUNNING MECHANICS

Without going into too much detail, remember that a stride has two phases: the stance phase (from the foot's contact with the ground until it leaves the ground) and the swing phase. During the stance phase, the pelvis moves above the entire propulsion zone, going from behind, to above, and then in front of the foot.

The stance phase can be further divided into two parts:

➔ Absorption, which lasts from the moment the foot touches the ground until the pelvis moves directly above the foot. This deceleration phase includes the cushioning of the fall of the center of gravity and control of the weight until the next phase.

➔ Propulsion, which lasts from the moment the pelvis is over the foot until the foot leaves the ground. This part helps maintain the pace by driving the pelvis forward.

As for the swing phase, it also has two components:

➔ First, the initial swing, or the travel of the leg from behind the pelvis to the point where it crosses the knee under the hips. This component includes the bending of the knee that lifts the foot toward the buttocks.

➔ Then, the terminal swing, which lasts from the meeting of the knees until the foot touches the ground. This is the front travel portion of the free leg; the thigh lifts, pointing the knee to the front, as high as the running speed is fast (a sprinter lifts the thigh to almost horizontal). Then the knee bends so that the foot can land on the ground.

The movement of the upper body is synchronized with the legs, always in contralateral opposition.
The trajectory of the upper body is the final point of both the forward motion and the backward motion. The arms pass by the torso, and the elbows are at the lowest point of their trajectory.

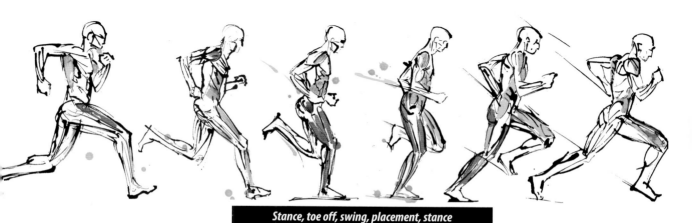

Stance, toe off, swing, placement, stance

PARAMETERS OF RUNNING

Just as you can calibrate the load in resistance training, for example, in weight or in tempo, you can use parameters in running to focus your work to make progress in a certain area. You can use speed, of course, but speed is not infinitely adjustable, and it is influenced by both stride amplitude and frequency. Those are the elements we strive to improve through physical and technical training as a way to increase running speed. Speed is a product of stride length and the number of strides over a certain length of time.

In fact, if you know the number of steps over a given distance for a given time, you can easily calculate the average amplitude and step frequency as well as average speed. Although at first an increase in amplitude may decrease the step frequency, the goal of physical and technical training is to increase the amplitude while preserving the initial frequency.

The second parameter is the time spent in contact and in swing. As speed increases, contact time decreases. To be efficient, you need to "scratch" the floor as quickly as possible and, above all, avoid "crashing" each time you land.

Finally, you need to consider the trajectory of the pelvis. To increase your speed, you have to keep your center of gravity from rising with each landing, smooth out its trajectory, and decrease the time spent in the swing phase.

Technique tips

- The center of gravity should move linearly.
- The pelvis tilts backward.
- The arms and legs are synchronized contralaterally.
- The torso is erect.
- The weight should be on the front of the foot.
- The stride amplitude increases without a decrease in the step frequency.

1. Concentric phase

The front of the thigh is working the hardest.

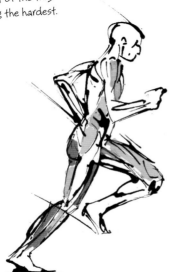

2. Eccentric phase

The back of the thigh is working the hardest.

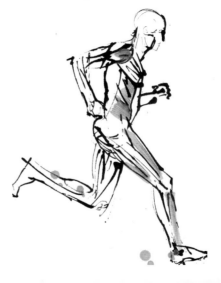

✖ MECHANICS OF STRIDE ADAPTATION

The requirements for running vary depending on the workout, but optimal stride mechanics differ depending on the distance being run. A video analysis of runners' leg movements has shown what the best runners in the world do in each of their specialties, and models of these movements have been created. These models are sometimes called *poulaines*, because the leg movements really do resemble these pointed shoes from the Middle Ages. Using the ear as a fixed point (not the hip, which is mobile) and the tip of the toe as a focal point for the trajectory of the feet, we can make <u>the following model</u>. The longer the race (and so the more moderate the pace), the higher the back cycle of the legs will be (like the heel of a shoe). Conversely, the front cycle (the toe of the shoe) gets larger as running speed increases. <u>On the following page we show you the ideal foot trajectories for a few specialties.</u>

→ See the drawing below.

→ See the drawings on the next page.

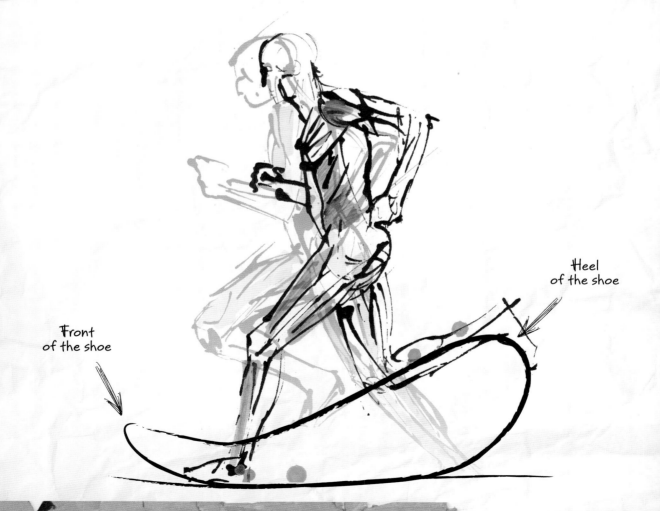

Heel of the shoe

Front of the shoe

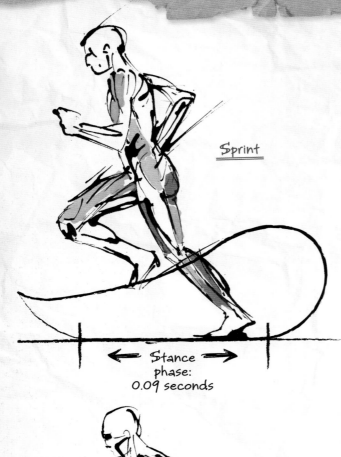

Sprint

← Stance →
phase:
0.09 seconds

The relationship between shoe shape and intensity

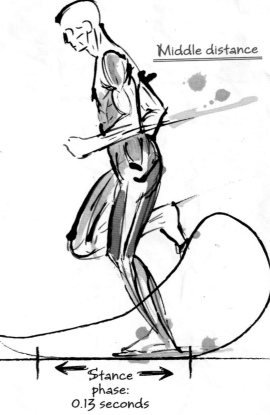

Middle distance

← Stance →
phase:
0.13 seconds

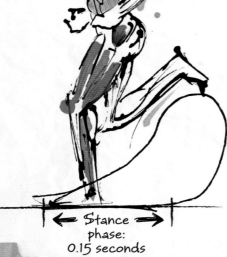

Long distance

← Stance →
phase:
0.15 seconds

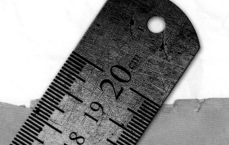

Here are a few technical drills to improve running technique. You can use them as a warm-up later:

- Unilateral heels to butt
- Raising one knee
- Running backward

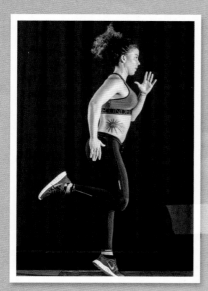

Heels to butt

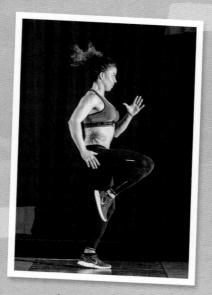

Raising the knee

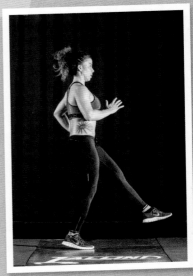

Running backward

Should you wear minimalist shoes?

Minimalist shoes have invaded gyms and clubs because they are as useful in weightlifting (especially because they use more of the plantar contraction reflexes on the ground) as they are in running. The virtues of these shoes are real; they provide sensation feedback to athletes and promote natural movement. Still, be careful and remember that you have been walking in shoes (often cushioned shoes) forever. You also learned to run in these cushioned shoes. These running shoes did not just have a tiny cushion; they were often equipped with thick cushions. Finally, remember that although minimalist shoes increase sensations, they also increase the impact and therefore do not spare your bones and joints. If you want to run greater distances, you must pace yourself. Lastly, minimalist shoes can disturb motor movements so much that, beyond the risk of injury caused by running with bad form, the small amount of energy spent in carefully managing your weight may well deceive you.

We think the best strategy is to compromise. First, introduce new shoes gradually; you should not go from old shoes one day to new shoes the next day. This has nothing to do with training; it is just common sense.

Then you can alternate shoes to enjoy the pleasures and mitigate the risks.
Ideally, you will choose the pair best suited for the workout.

- Workout combining weightlifting and short-distance running: minimalist shoes or multisport running shoes
- Low intensity floor work: running shoes with gel cushion or a trial period with minimalist shoes
- Predominantly weightlifting: weightlifting shoes with wooden soles
- Workouts with intermittent running: running shoes with gel cushion
- Multistation circuit workout: multisport running shoes or minimalist shoes

WORKOUT – RUNNING

WORKOUT 1 – DOUBLES AND HALVES

45 SECONDS OF RUNNING, 45 SECONDS OF RECOVERY
1 MINUTE 30 SECONDS OF RUNNING, 1 MINUTE 30 SECONDS OF RECOVERY
3 MINUTES OF RUNNING, 3 MINUTES OF RECOVERY
6 MINUTES OF RUNNING, 6 MINUTES OF RECOVERY
3 MINUTES OF RUNNING, 3 MINUTES OF RECOVERY
1 MINUTE 30 SECONDS OF RUNNING, 1 MINUTE 30 SECONDS OF RECOVERY
45 SECONDS OF RUNNING, 45 SECONDS OF RECOVERY

WORKOUT 2 – DEMANDING 60

1 MINUTE OF RUNNING FOR EACH SET. RECOVERY STARTS AT 1 MINUTE AND THEN DECREASES BY 10 SECONDS FOR EVERY SET. WHEN THERE ARE ONLY 10 SECONDS LEFT, THE RECOVERY TIME INCREASES BY 10 SECONDS EVERY SET.

1 MINUTE OF RUNNING, 1 MINUTE OF RECOVERY
1 MINUTE OF RUNNING, 50 SECONDS OF RECOVERY
1 MINUTE OF RUNNING, 40 SECONDS OF RECOVERY
1 MINUTE OF RUNNING, 30 SECONDS OF RECOVERY
1 MINUTE OF RUNNING, 20 SECONDS OF RECOVERY
1 MINUTE OF RUNNING, 10 SECONDS OF RECOVERY
1 MINUTE OF RUNNING, 20 SECONDS OF RECOVERY
1 MINUTE OF RUNNING, 30 SECONDS OF RECOVERY
1 MINUTE OF RUNNING, 40 SECONDS OF RECOVERY
1 MINUTE OF RUNNING, 50 SECONDS OF RECOVERY
1 MINUTE OF RUNNING, 1 MINUTE OF RECOVERY

WORKOUT 3 – TEQUILA SHOT

3 X 10-METER SPRINT, 30 SECONDS OF RECOVERY
3 X 30-METER SPRINT, 30 SECONDS OF RECOVERY
3 X 50-METER SPRINT, 30 SECONDS OF RECOVERY,
30-METER SPRINT, 1 MINUTE OF RECOVERY
3 X 10-METER SPRINT, 30 SECONDS OF RECOVERY
3 X 30-METER SPRINT, 30 SECONDS OF RECOVERY
3 X 50-METER SPRINT, 30 SECONDS OF RECOVERY,
30-METER SPRINT, 1 MINUTE OF RECOVERY

The golden rule of one too many reps

The Modern Art of High Intensity Training was created out of an anatomical demand, a view of training in which proper form—the heart of injury prevention—is never compromised. Never make the mistake of continuing a set to the point where you have to cheat on your technique. When your form deteriorates, stop the set

THE 15-WEEK MODERN ART PROGRAM

200   Phase 1–Fundamentals

202   Phase 2–Structural Development

204   Phase 3–Intensify

206   Phase 4–Optimize

Chapter 3

Phase 1, fundamentals: Metabolic endurance and cardiovascular endurance, fundamental skill and technique development (3 weeks)

Phase 2, structural development: Functional hypertrophy (5 weeks)

Phase 3, intensify: Strength development and intensification of endurance (maximum aerobic power) (4 weeks)

Phase 4, optimize: Muscle power and endurance (3 weeks)

✱ PHASE 1 - FUNDAMENTALS

Day	1	2	3	4	5	6	7
Workout	Snatch instruction Squats 4 x 9 (p. 89) Renegade push-ups 4 x 10 (p. 162) <u>Workout</u> 3 to 6 rounds: -6 kettle-bell swings (p. 128) -6 air squats -6 sit-ups -6 pull-ups (p. 143) -6 forward lunges (p. 140)	Kettle-bell clean instruction <u>Workout</u> 20 min nonstop with light kettlebell: -20 swings (p. 128) -20 V-ups (p. 182) -20 goblet squats (p. 98) -20 straight-leg deadlifts (p. 136) -20 alterna-ting cleans (p. 34)	Low intensity run 7 km	Clean instruction Deadlifts (p. 125) 4 x 9 Pull-ups (p. 143) 4 x 10 <u>Workout</u> As many times as possible in 15 min: -200 m run -10 V-ups (p. 182)	Low intensity run 7 km	Technique workout Sandbag cleans 3 x 10 (p. 54) Thrusters 3 x 10 (p. 103) Bench presses 3 x 10 (p. 120) Overhead squats 3 x 10 (p. 100) 3 rope climbs (p. 154)	Rest

Day	8	9	10	11	12	13	14
Workout	Snatch instruction Squats 5 x 7 (p. 89) Workout Every min for 15 min: -2 deadlifts (p. 125) -1 snatch (p. 60) End with 10 min of varied core work	Kettle-bell clean instruction Workout 1 10 min nonstop: -10 alternating kettle-bell swings (p. 128) -10 kettle-bell thrusters (p. 103) -10 alternating kettle-bell lunges (p. 140) Workout 2 10 min nonstop: -400 m run -1 rope climb (4 m, p. 154) - 10 Turkish get-ups (5 on the right and 5 on the left, p. 187)	Rest	Clean instruction Sumo dead-lifts 5 x 7 (p. 138) Workout As many times as possible in 20 min: -200 m run -10 V-ups (p. 182) -10 straight-leg deadlifts (p. 136)	Low intensity run 10 km	Muscle-up technique 3 rope climbs (p. 154) Workout 6 rounds: -10 rene-gade push-ups (p. 162) -20 pull-ups using a band (p. 143) End with 4 x 10 barbell ab rollouts (p. 190)	Low intensity run 6 km

Day	15	16	17	18	19	20	21
Workout	Rest	Low intensity run 7 km	Rest	Weightlifting instruction Overhead squats 3 x 7 (p. 100) Cleans 4 x 3 (p. 34) Snatches 3 x 3 (p. 60) Workout 10 min nonstop run, then 12 x 30 sec of intense running alternated with 30 sec of rest	Rest	Sustained-intensity run 5 km	Rest

✖ PHASE 2 - STRUCTURAL DEVELOPMENT

Day	22	23	24	25	26	27	28
Workout	Overhead squats 3 x 10 (p. 100) 4 squats (at your 8-rep max, p. 89) Recovery: 90 sec 4 bench presses (at your 8-rep max, p. 120) Recovery: 90 sec Workout As many times as possible in 5 min: -10 kettlebell swings (p. 128) -10 burpees (p. 165) -50 m sprint -10 knee tuck jumps 2 rounds, 4 min recovery	Core exercise circuit: -10 barbell ab rollouts (p. 190) -10 V-ups (p. 182) -30 sec elbow plank -10 back extensions Workout As many sets as necessary, as fast as possible: -200 push-ups (p. 158) -300 air squats (p. 89) -100 pull-ups (p. 143) -200 sit-ups -300 air squats	Rest	Renegade push-ups 3 x 10 (p. 162) 4 x deadlifts (at your 8-rep max, p. 125) Recovery: 90 sec 4 x bent-over rows (at your 8-rep max, p. 83) Recovery: 90 sec Workout Every min for 6 min, as fast as possible: -5 complete burpees (p. 165) -60 m sprint -5 kettle-bell thrusters (p. 103) -6 V-ups (p. 182) 2 rounds, 4 min recovery	Rest	6 sets: 30 sec plank, 10 overhead squats (p.100) Recovery: 1 min Workout -As many push-ups (p. 158) as possible in 5 min -As many squats (p. 89) at 75% of maximum as possible in 2 min -As many pull-ups (p. 143) as possible in 5 min -As many thrusters (p. 103) at 75% of maximum as possible in 2 min	Snatches 3 x 3 (p. 60) 4 x front squats (at your 8-rep max, p. 97) Recovery: 90 sec 4 x narrow grip bench presses (at your 8-rep max, p. 120) Recovery: 90 sec Workout As fast as possible: -3 snatches (p. 60) -10 tire flips (p. 56) -10 complete burpees (p. 165) -3 tire flips -50 m sprint 3 rounds, 3 min recovery

Day	29	30	31	32	33	34	35
Workout	4 or 5 rounds: -Front squats (at your 5-rep max, p. 97) -Recovery: 10 sec -Squats (at your 5-rep max, p. 89) -Recovery: 2 min -6 knee tuck jumps -Recovery: 2 min Workout 5 rounds as fast as possible: -8 deadlifts (p. 125) at 50% of maximum -50 m run -8 complete burpees (p. 165) -50 m run -8 knee tuck jumps -50 m run	Rest	4 or 5 rounds: -Shoulder-width grip bench press (at your 5-rep max, p. 120) -Recovery: 10 sec -Wide-grip bench press (at your 5-rep max, p. 120) - Recovery: 2 min -6 explosive push-ups (your choice, p. 169) -Recovery: 2 min Workout As many rounds as possible in 12 min: -10 kettlebell snatches (p. 76) -20 kettlebell swings (p. 128) -10 sit-ups	Squats 4 x 5 (p. 89) Clean and jerks 4 x 3 (p. 34) Hang cleans 4 x 3 Workout Every min for 7 min: -Clean (p. 34) -Squat (p. 89) -Jerk (p. 47)	Rest	Run 4 km Workout -10 x 30 sec of fast running -30 sec of slow running -3 min rest 10 x 30 sec fast running -30 sec rest Run 1 km as active recovery	4 or 5 rounds: -Front squats (at your 5-rep max, p. 97) -Recovery: 10 sec -Squats (at your 5-rep max, p. 89) -Recovery: 2 min -6 knee tuck jumps -Recovery: 2 min Workout 5 rounds as fast as possible: -8 pull-ups (p. 143) -10 land-mine thrusters (p. 115) -10 pull-ups -20 landmine obliques (p. 117) -10 pull-ups

Day	36	37	38	39	40	41	42
Workout	Run 3 km Workout Alternate fast running and active recovery in a pyramid: -15, 15 -30, 30 -45, 45 -60, 60 -45, 45 -30, 30 -15, 15 2 rounds, 2 min of rest between rounds End with 1 km of running to recover	Rest	Overhead squats 3 x 10 (p. 100) 4 x squats (at your max for failure at 7 to 9 reps, p. 89) Recovery: 2 min 4 x supersets: -8 thrusters (p. 103) -8 bench presses (p. 120) -8 push-ups (p. 158) 3 rounds, 1 min of recovery Workout Combine in 6 rounds: -1 snatch (p. 60) -10 box jumps -As many pull-ups as possible (p. 143)	3 rope climbs (p. 154) alternated with 10 air squats (p. 89) Workout Do 25 reps in less than 2 min at 75% of maximum: -Deadlifts (p. 125) -Weighted pull-ups (p. 143) -Lunges to the right and then to the left (p. 140) -Bent-over rows (p. 83)	Rest	Cleans 3 x 6 (p. 34) 4 x deadlifts (at your max for failure at 7 to 9 reps, p. 123) Recovery: 2 min 4 x supersets: -8 pull-ups (p. 143) -8 bent-over rows (p. 83) -8 renegade push-up, row, and press combination (p. 162) 3 rounds, 1 min of recovery Workout -400 air squats (p. 89) -300 complete burpees (p. 165) -200 push-ups (p. 158) -100 arabesques (p. 134) -50 pull-ups (p. 143)	Rest

Day	43	44	45	46	47	48	49
Workout	Rest	4 or 5 rounds: -Front squats (at your 5-rep max, p. 97) -Recovery: 10 sec -Squats (at your 5-rep max, p.89) -Recovery: 2 min -6 knee tuck jumps -Recovery: 2 min Workout 5 rounds as fast as possible: -8 clapping push-ups (p. 167) -10 box jumps -8 complete burpees (p. 165) -10 box jumps -8 bent-over rows (p. 83) -50 m run	Run 3 km Workout 5 x 2 min fast running, 2 min active recovery 10 x 30-30 15 x 15-15	Rest	4 or 5 rounds: -Weighted pull-ups on the rings (at your 5-rep max, p. 143) -Recovery: 10 sec -Bent-over rows (at your 5-rep max, p. 83) -Recovery: 2 min -6 clapping pull-ups (p. 148) -Recovery: 2 min Workout -20 kettle-bell thrusters (p. 103) -20 V-ups (p. 182) -Then 18, 15, 12, 9, 5, 3, 1	Run 4 km Workout 8 x 2 min fast running, 2 min active recovery 5 x 30-30 10 x 15-15 2 x 2-2	Rest

Day	50	51	52	53	54	55	56
Workout	Rest	Moderate-intensity run 7 km	Rest	Weightlifting instruction Overhead squats 3 x 7 (p. 100) Cleans 4 x 3 (p. 34) Snatches 3 x 3 (p. 60) Workout 10 min of nonstop running Then 12 x 30 sec of intense running alternated with 30 sec of rest	Rest	Sustained-intensity run 5 km	Rest

✖ PHASE 3 - INTENSIFY

Day	57	58	59	60	61	62	63
Workout	Clean and jerks 5 x 3 (p. 34) Hang cleans 3 x 3 Workout 5 rounds: 1 clean at 65% of maximum and 1 knee tuck jumps for 1 min, then recover for 3 min	Max deadlifts 4 x 5 (p. 125) Shoulder-width bench press 4 x 5 (p. 120) Pyramid: -200 m sprint in each set -1 min recovery -Subtract 10 sec of rest each set -When only 10 sec are left, add 10 sec to each set until you get back to 1 min	Rest	Snatches 5 x 3 (p. 60) Snatches from the thighs, 3 x 3 Workout 5 rounds: 1 snatch at 65% of maximum and 1 shuttle sprint 5 + 5 m for 1 min, then recover for 3 min	Max squats 4 x 5 (p. 89) Bent-over rows 4 x 5 (p. 83) Sustained-intensity run 5 km	Rest	Rest

Day	64	65	66	67	68	69	70
Workout	Clean and jerks 5 x 2 (p. 34) Deadlifts 5 x 4 (p. 125) <u>Workout</u> -10 cleans at 40% of maximum -400 m run 6 rounds, 1 min recovery	Snatches 5 x 2 (p. 60) Shoulder-width bench press 5 x 4 (p. 120) <u>Workout</u> As many times as possible in 2 min at 40% of maximum: -10 snatches -10 overhead squats (p. 100) -10 burpees (p. 165) 6 rounds, 1 min recovery	Rest	Hang cleans 5 x 2 Squats 5 x 4 (p. 89) <u>Workout</u> At 40% of maximum: -6 clean and jerks (p. 34) -200 m row 6 rounds, 1 min recovery	Snatches from the thighs 5 x 2 Bent-over rows 5 x 4 (p. 83) <u>Workout</u> As many times as possible in 2 min at 40% of maximum: -10 kettlebell swings (p. 128) -10 thrusters (p. 103) -10 knee tuck jumps 6 rounds, 1 min recovery	Sustained-intensity run 2 x 3 km	Rest

Day	71	72	73	74	75	76	77
Workout	Clean and jerks 6 x 1 (p. 34) Explosive thrusters 5 x 2 (p. 103) <u>Workout</u> -1 clean and jerk -10 box jumps -10 thrusters at 50% of maximum -100 m sprint 10 rounds, 1 min recovery	Find your 1-rep max in squats (p. 89) and bent-over rows (p. 83) in less than 15 min <u>Workout</u> -10 complete burpees (p. 165) -10 battle rope waves (p. 174) -150 m sprint -10 box jumps -10 knee tuck jumps -150 m sprint 8 rounds, 1 min recovery	Rest	Snatches 6 x 1 (p. 60) Explosive thrusters 5 x 2 (p. 103) <u>Workout</u> -1 snatch lunge (p. 140) -10 jumping lunges (p. 141) -10 max vertical jumps -100 m row 10 rounds, 1 min recovery	Find your 1-rep max in deadlift (p. 125) and bench press (p. 120) in less than 15 min <u>Workout</u> -10 thrusters (p. 103) -10 landmine obliques (p. 117) -100 m sprint -10 knee tuck jumps -10 landmine thrusters -100 m sprint 8 rounds, 1 min recovery	Sustained-intensity run 2 x 3 km	Rest

Day	78	79	80	81	82	83	84
Workout	Clean and jerks 6 x 1 (p. 34) Explosive thrusters 5 x 2 (p. 103) Workout 10 rounds: -5 deadlifts at 70% of maximum (p. 125) -5 barbell ab rollouts (p. 190) -10 box jumps -10 V-ups (p. 182) Max rest: 1 min	Find your 1-rep max in squats (p. 89) and bent-over rows (p. 83) in less than 15 min Workout Every min for 10 min: -1 snatch (p. 60) -1 bent-over row (p. 83) -1 barbell ab rollout (p. 190) Then 5 rounds: -5 dynamic, light snatches -7 squats (p. 89) -4 double knee tuck push-ups (p. 169)	Rest	Snatches 6 x 1 (p. 60) Explosive thrusters 5 x 2 (p. 103) Workout As many as possible in 20 min: -5 dynamic bench presses at 70% of maximum (p. 120) -5 bench jumps -10 complete burpees (p. 165) -10 V-ups (p. 182) Max rest: 1 min	Rest	Find your 1-rep max for deadlift (p. 125) and bench press (p. 120) in less than 15 min Workout Every min for 10 min: -1 clean (p. 34) -1 squat (p. 89) -1 bent-over row (p. 83) -1 deadlift (p. 125)	Rest

✖ PHASE 4 - OPTIMIZE

Day	85	86	87	88	89	90	91
Workout	Snatches 2 x 3 (p. 60) Squats 3 x 3 (p. 89) 30 sec rest, 4 knee tuck jumps Workout Every min for 10 min: -1 snatch -4 box jumps -20 m sprint Every min for 10 min: -1 snatch -4 clapping pull-ups (p. 148) -20 m sprint	Deadlifts 2 x 5 (p. 125) Weighted pull-ups 3 x 3 (p. 143) 30 sec rest 1 rope climb 5 m (p. 154) Workout Every min for 5 min: -3 deadlifts -1 clean (p. 34) -2 jerks (p. 47) -2 cleans -2 squats (p. 89) -2 jerks 7 rounds in 10 min	Rest	Cleans 2 x 3 (p. 34) Bench press 3 x 3 (p. 120) 30 sec rest 3 clapping push-ups (p. 167) Workout Every min for 10 min: -1 clean -5 burpees (p. 165) -30 m shuttle sprint Every min for 10 min: -1 clean -4 Aztec push-ups (p. 171) -20 m sprint	Rest	10 sets, 2 min recovery: -3 cleans (p. 34) -40 m sprint -1 clean -20 m sprint 10 sets, 2 min recovery: -3 snatches (p. 60) -6 box jumps -1 snatch -3 box jumps	Rest

Day	92	93	94	95	96	97	98
Workout	Strength: 2 heavy clean and jerks (p. 34) 3 light clean and jerks Workout 10 rounds: -5 landmine squats at 70% of maximum (p. 115) -5 barbell ab rollouts (p. 190) -10 burpees (p. 165) -10 toes to bar (p. 185)	Strength: 3 heavy bent-over rows (p. 83) 4 light bent-over rows Do 6 sets Workout 4 rounds: -As many deadlifts as possible in 1 min (p. 125) -Recover for 1 min -As many abdominal exercises as possible in 1 min -Recover for 1 min -As many push-ups as possible in 1 min (p. 158) -Recover for 1 min	-3 heavy squats (p. 89) -4 light squats Do 6 sets Workout -7 sets of 6 clapping pull-ups (p. 148) -50 m sprint Recovery: 4 min	Rest	-3 heavy cleans (p. 34) -4 light cleans Do 6 sets Workout 3 rounds of this circuit as fast as possible: -8 tire flips (p. 56) -20 complete burpees (p. 165) -6 clapping pull-ups (p. 148) -400 m run	-3 heavy bench presses (p. 120) -4 light bench presses Do 6 sets Workout 3 rounds: -As many bar squats as possible in 1 min (p. 89) -Recover for 1 min -As many abdominal exercises as possible in 1 min -Recover for 1 min -As many pull-ups as possible in 1 min (p. 143) -Recover for 1 min	Strength: 3 heavy deadlifts (p. 125) 4 light deadlifts Do 6 sets Workout -7 sets of 6 double knee tuck push-ups (p. 169) -50 m sprint Recovery: 4 min

Day	99	100	101	102	103	104	105
Workout	Rest	Snatches 6 x 6 with max power (p. 60), recovery: 2 min Workout Do 4 rounds as fast as possible: -3 squats (p. 89) -6 box jumps -6 knee tuck jumps -3 squats	Bent-over rows 6 x 6 with max power (p. 83), recovery: 2 min Workout -21, 15, 9 reps of bench press (p. 120) -Complete burpees (p. 165) -Renegade rows (p. 162) -Then as many pull-ups as possible in 5 min (p. 143)	Squats 6 x 6 with max power, recovery: 2 min Workout 10 x 30 m sprint starting every min	Rest	Clean and jerks 6 x 6 (p. 34) Workout Do 4 rounds as fast as possible: -3 deadlifts (p. 125) -6 vertical jumps -6 knee tuck jumps -3 deadlifts	Bench press 6 x 6 with max power (p. 120), recovery: 2 min Workout -21, 15, 9 reps of goblet squats (p. 98) -Side jumps onto a bench -Dips (p. 180)

BIBLIOGRAPHY

Aubert, F., Chauffin, T. (2007). Athlétisme 3. Les courses. *Ed. Revue EPS*, 15–84.

Bergh, U., Ekblom, B. (1979). Influence of muscle temperature on maximal strength and power output in human muscle. *Acta. Physiol. Scand.* 107: 332–337.

Bishop, D., Edge, J., Mendez-Villanueva, A., Thomas, C., Schneiker, K. (September 2009). High-intensity exercise decreases muscle buffer capacity via a decrease in protein buffering in human skeletal muscle. *Pflugers Arch.* 458 (5): 929–36.

Bolliet, O. (2013). *Approche moderne du développement de la force.* Ed 4Trainer, 1st ed.

Brooks, G.A. (2000). Intra- and extra-cellular lactate shuttles. *Med. Sci. Sports Exerc.* 32:790–799.

Broussal-Derval, A., Bolliet O. (2012). *La préparation physique moderne.* Ed 4Trainer, 2nd ed., 117–121.

Bryanton, M.A., Kennedy, M.D., Carey, J.P., Chiu, L.Z. (October 2012). Effect of squat depth and barbell load on relative muscular effort in squatting, *J. Strength Cond. Res.* 26 (10): 2820–2828.

Cadore, E.L., Izquierdo, M. (August 2013). New strategies for the concurrent strength-, power-, and endurance-training prescription in elderly individuals. *J Am. Med. Dir. Assoc.* 14 (8): 623–624.

Coffey, G., Hawley, A. (2007). The molecular bases of training adaptation. *Sports Med.* 37 (9): 737–763.

Choi, D., Cole, K.J., Goodpaster, B.H., Fink, W.J., Costill, D.L. (August 1994). Effect of passive and active recovery on the resynthesis of muscle glycogen. *Med. Sci. Sports Exerc.* 26 (8): 992–996.

Cornu, C. (2002). Le Cross Training: de la compétition à l'entretien physique. *Sport, Santé et Préparation Physique* 3:6–7.

Davitt, P.M., Pellegrino, J., Schanzer, J., Tjionas, H., Arent, S.M. (July 2014). The effects of a combined resistance training and endurance exercise program in inactive college females: Does order matter? *J. Strength Cond. Res.* 28 (7): 1937–1945.

Docherty, D., Sporer, B. (December 2000). A proposed model for examining the interference phenomenon between concurrent aerobic and strength training. *Sports Med.* 30 (6): 385–394.

Edge, J., Eynon, N., McKenna, M.J., Goodman, C.A., Harris, R.C., Bishop, D.J. (February 2013). Altering the rest interval during high-intensity interval training does not affect muscle or performance adaptations. *Exp. Physiol.* 98 (2): 481–90.

Esformes, J.I., Bampouras, T.M. (November 2013). Effect of back squat depth on lower body post-activation potentiation. *J. Strength Cond. Res.* 27 (11): 2997–3000.

Ferrari, R., Kruel, L.F.M., Cadore, E.L., Alberton, C.L., Izquierdo, M., Conceição, M., Pinto, R.S., Radaelli, R., Wilhelm, E., Bottaro, M., Ribeiro, J.P., (November 2013). Efficiency of twice weekly concurrent training in trained elderly men. *Exp. Gerontol.* 48 (11): 1236–1242.

Flynn, M.G., Carroll, K.K., Hall, H.L., Bushman, B.A., Brolinson, P.G., Weideman, C.A., (1998). Cross training: Indices of training stress and performance. *Med. Sci. Sports Exer.* 30 (2), 294–300.

Fry, A.C., Smith, J. C., Schilling, B.K. (November 2003). Effect of knee position on hip and knee torques during the barbell squat. *J. Strength Cond. Res.* 17 (4): 629–633.

Garcia-Pallares, J., Sanchez-Medina, L., Carrasco, L., Diaz, A., Izquierdo, M. (2009). Endurance and neuromuscular changes in world-class level kayakers during a periodized training cycle. *Eur. J. Appl. Physiol.* 106 (4): 629–638.

Glaister, M. (2005). Multiple sprint work: Physiological responses, mechanisms of fatigue and the influence of aerobic fitness. *Sports Med.* 35 (9) 757–777.

Gullett, J.C., Tillman, M.D., Gutierrez, G.M., Chow, J.W., (2009). A biomechanical comparison of back and front squats in healthy trained individuals. *J. Strength Cond. Res.* 23 (1): 284–292.

Impellizzeri, F.M., Marcora, S.M., Rampinini, E., Mognoni, P., Sassi, A. (2005). Correlations between physiological variables and performance in high level cross country off road cyclists. *Br. J. Sports Med.* 39:747–751.

Izquierdo, M., Exposito, R.J., Garcia-Pallare, J., Medina, L., Villareal, E., (June 2010). Concurrent endurance and strength training not to failure optimizes performance gains. *Med. Sci. Sports Exerc.* 42 (6): 1191–1199.

Jones, T.W., Howatson, G., Russell, M., French, D.N. (December 2013). Performance and neuromuscular adaptations following differing ratios of concurrent strength and endurance training. *J. Strength Cond. Res.* 27 (12): 3342–3351.

Juel, C. (1996). Lactate/proton co-transport in skeletal muscle: regulation and importance for pH homeostasis. *Acta Physiol. Scand.* 156:69–374.

Khosravi, M., Tayebi, S.M., Safari, H. (April 2013). Single and concurrent effects of endurance and resistance training on pulmonary function. *Iran J. Basic Med. Sci.* 16 (4): 628–34.

Lacour, J.R., Bouvat, E., Barthélémy, J.C. (1990). Post-competition blood lactate concentrations as indicators of anaerobic energy expenditure during 400-m and 800-m races. *Eur. J. Appl. Physiol. Occup. Physiol.* 61 (3–4): 172–176.

Massey, C., Vincent, J., Maneval, M., Johnson, J.T. (May 2005). Influence of range of motion in resistance training in women: Early phase adaptations. *J. Strength Cond. Res.* 19 (2): 409–411.

McBride, J.M., Kirby, T.J., Haines, T.L., Skinner, J.W., Delalija, A. (March 2011). Relationship between impulse, peak force and jump squat performance with variation in loading and squat depth. *J. Strength Cond. Res.* 25.

Mendez-Villanueva, A., Edge, J., Suriano, R., Hamer, P., Bishop, D. (2012). The recovery of repeated-sprint exercise is associated with PCr resynthesis, while muscle pH and EMG amplitude remain depressed. *PLoS One.* 7 (12): e51977.

Miller, B.F., Fattor, J.A., Jacobs, K.A., Horning, M.A., Navazio, F., Lindinger, M.I., Brooks, G.A. (2002). Lactate and glucose interactions during rest and exercise in men: Effect of exogenous lactate infusion. *J. Physiol.* 544 (Pt 3): 963–975.

Millet, G.-Y., Lepers, R. (2004). Alterations of neuromuscular function after prolonged running, cycling and skiing exercises. *Sports Med.* 34 (2): 105–16.

Poortmans, J.R. (2003). *Biochimie des activités physiques*. De Boeck Université.

Radlinger, L., Bachmann, W., Homburg, J., Leuenberger, U., Thaddey, G. (Eds.). (1998). Methoden des Krafttrainings. In: *Rehabilitatives krafttraining*. Stuttgart; New York: Thieme. 49–87.

Robergs, R.A., Ghiasvand, F., Parker, D. (September 2004). Biochemistry of exercise-induced metabolic acidosis. *Am. J. Physiol. Regul. Integr. Comp. Physiol.* 287 (3): R502–R516.

Salem, G.J., Powers, C.M. (2001). Patellofemoral joint kinetics during squatting in collegiate women athletes. *Clinical Biomechanics* 16 (5): 424–430.

Schmidt, R.F., Thews, G. (Eds.). (2013). *Physiologie des menschen*. Springer-Verlag.

Sedano, S., Marín, P.J., Cuadrado, G., Redondo, J.C. (September 2013). Concurrent training in elite male runners: the influence of strength versus muscular endurance training on performance outcomes. *J. Strength Cond. Res.* 27 (9): 2433–2443.

Signorile, J.F., Weber, B., Roll, B., Caruso, J.F., Lowensteyn, I., Perry, A.C. (August 1994). An electromyographical comparison of the squat and knee extension exercises. *J. Strength Cond. Res.* 8 (3): 178–183.

Schwanbeck, S., Chilibeck, P.D., Binsted, G. (December 2009). A comparison of free weight squat to smith machine squat using electromyography. *J. Strength Cond. Res.* 23 (9): 2588–2591.

Schwellnus, M., Drew, N., Collins, M. (2008). Muscle cramping in athletes—risk factors, clinical assessment, and management. *Clin. Sports Med.* 27: 183–194.

Spencer, M., Bishop, D., Dawson, B., Goodman, C., Duffield, R. (2006). Metabolism and performance in repeated cycle sprints: Active versus passive recovery. *Med. Sci. Sports Exerc.* 38 (8): 1492–1499.

Stoboy, H. (1972). Neuromuskuläre funktion und körperliche leistung. In *Zentrale themen der sportmedizin*. Springer Berlin Heidelberg, 17-43.

Tanaka, H. (1994). Effects of cross-training. Transfer of training effects on V̇O2max between cycling, running and swimming. *Sports Med.* 18 (5): 330–339.

Thomas, C., Bishop, D.J., Lambert, K., Mercier, J., Brooks, G.A. (2012). Effects of acute and chronic exercise on sarcolemmal MCT1 and MCT4 contents in human skeletal muscles: Current status. *Am. J. Physiol. Regul. Integr. Comp. Physiol.* 302 (1): R1–R14.

Thibaudeau, C. (2007). Principe 4: S'entrainer jusqu'à l'échec musculaire positif. *Musculation à haut seuil d'activation*. 37–42.

Thibaudeau, C. (2007). Chapitre 6: Variables aiguës d'entraînement, point 3: Nombre de séries par groupe musculaire, *Le livre noir des secrets d'entraînement*. 72.

Weeks, C., Trevino, J., Blanchard, G., Kimpel, S. (March 2011). Effect of squat depth training on vertical jump performance. *J. Strength Cond. Res.* 25.

Wilson, G.J., Newton, R.U., Murphy, A.J., Humphries, B.J. (1993). The optimal training load for the development of dynamic athletic performance. *Med. Sci. Sports Exerc.* 25 (11): 1279–1286.

Zatsiorsky, V. (1995). *Science and practice of strength training*. Champaign, IL: Human Kinetics.

AURÉLIEN BROUSSAL-DERVAL

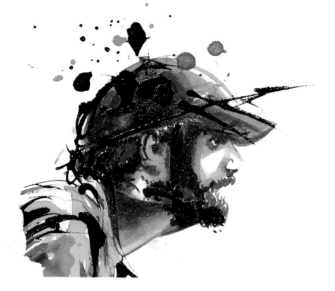

I have been interested in high intensity training since almost the beginning of my career in the 2000s.

As an athletic trainer in various sports in countries such as Russia, Spain, and Great Britain, I have worked with many high-level athletes who entrusted me to help them prepare. Naturally, the many influences and complex requirements of these athletes led me to incorporate weightlifting, athletic, and gymnastic content into my programs.

Given the explosion in popularity of these practices, I decided to compile the fruits of my experience and my abilities into a book for practitioners of all sports.

Aurélien Broussal-Derval holds a master's degree in physical, mental, and return-to-sport conditioning and a master's in engineering performance. He holds a one-year postgraduate degree in training with high-level training specialty from the National Institute of Sport and Physical Education (INSEP), and is a professor of sport. He is not only an academic author of French language reference works about physical conditioning such as *La préparation physique moderne* and *Les tests de terrain* but also a teacher at numerous European universities as well as a physical educator on the ground. He has trained, among others, the Russian and English judo teams and the French boxing team. Most recently, he has been coordinating research and innovation for the French Volleyball Federation.

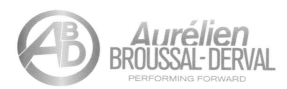

STÉPHANE GANNEAU

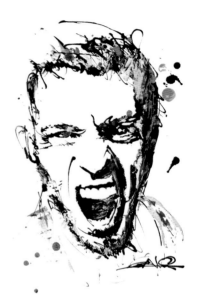

For some time, I have wanted to draw a series illustrating what is beneath the skin.

I was looking for a dynamic, intense medium to express the graphic style I had in mind.

Because I had been doing high intensity training for years to complement my judo training, this project was the perfect fusion of my two passions: sport and drawing.

Stéphane Ganneau is a designer for specialty trades in perfumes and cosmetics and is the author of several sport-marketing productions. A diligent and enlightened artist, he has been using his drawing abilities for sport illustrations for several years.

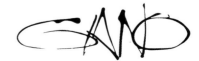

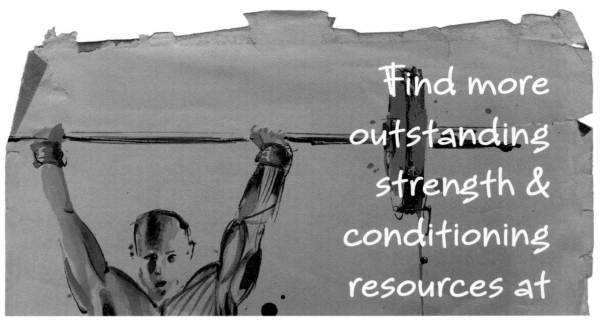
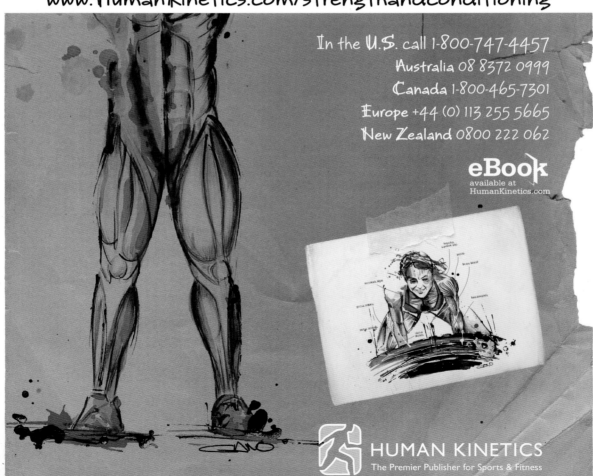